FIRM YOUR FANNY

Elizabeth Moreno

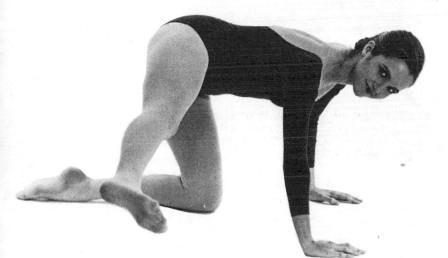

A PERIGEE BOOK

Perigee Books
are published by
G. P. Putnam's Sons
200 Madison Avenue
New York, New York 10016

Library of Congress Cataloging in Publication Data

Moreno, Elizabeth.
  Firm your fanny.

  (A. Perigee book)
  1. Reducing exercises. 2. Buttocks. I. Title.
RA781.6.M67   646.7′5   79-20065
ISBN 0-399-50462-1

First Perigee Printing, 1980
PRINTED IN THE UNITED STATES OF AMERICA

The Fanny

The fanny, according to Mr. Webster, is "A contraction of 'Aunt Fanny,' a fanciful euphemism for the buttocks." Whether you call it fanny, bottom, backside, derrière, or whatever, it is one of the most prominent parts of the body. Today we see it in tight French and western jeans and teenie-weenie bikinis. The sight can be pleasing or gross. Depending on your direction of approach, it forms either the first impression or the last, lingering image. There are very few that don't need firming. My aim here is to help you achieve the desired pear-shaped bottom, whether you are starting out as a basketball, a watermelon, or a gelatinous Mount McKinley.

The secretary's spread has become a chronic disease. Although women tend to carry their weight more on the hips and buttocks, many men find that they also need to tone up their haunches. They, as well as women, find themselves more and more inactive, whether it is in cars, at desks, or at business luncheons. Nature intended humans to provide for their fitness needs through physical labor and activity. But as we invent machines to work for us, our need for exercise has increased. The invention of the elevator, the car, and all other labor-saving devices has made our bodies victims of our leisure.

Looseness, sluggishness, and loss of tone come from disuse of buttocks muscles. Although the gluteus maximus, an often used synonym for the behind, is the best known and largest muscle (it is used to climb, run, and dance), there are other important muscles that make up the buttocks. The gluteus medius plays a role in correct posture; it keeps the hips level. It is also used for walking and running. Others, such as the gemellus inferior, the gemellus superior, the piriformis, the obturator internus, the obturator externus, and the quadratus femoris, are deep muscles which cause the leg to rotate in the hip socket and help move the thigh in different directions. The iliacus, the tensor fasciae, and the gluteus minimus also play an important part in all movements related to exercises for the buttocks area. In addition, there are many other muscles that are not actually part of the muscles of the buttocks area but aid in the execution of movements involving the fanny. Thus in order to activate the different muscles that make up the buttocks, different types of exercises are included. Some are meant primarily to reduce the size of the rump, others to trim and firm. Because these buttocks muscles are directly connected to other muscles in the body, you will feel some of the exercises working on the muscles in the inner thigh, the outer thigh, the back of the thigh, and on occasion the abdomen.

Unless you have medical problems and your doctor has forbidden it, you should exercise. If your physical activity must be limited, some of the basic exercises in this book will be easy to do. If you are already involved in a regular exercise program, this book can provide more intensive help for spot reducing in the backside area.

As a beginning, think about how you move. Do you let your buttocks just hang behind? *Don't let the fanny hang there . . . use it!* Inactivity and sedentary ways are the body's self-made enemies. If you are in good health use the stairs whenever possible instead of taking elevators. When you walk, try to feel how your leg moves from the hip socket. Use your gluteal muscles as you walk. If you stand on public transportation, practice moving with the motion of the bus in what I call the "Strap Hanger's Stance." On elevators, street corners, when the water for the bathtub is running and you are brushing your teeth, practice the "buttock squeeze." When doing housework or using the lower drawer of a filing cabinet, bend your knees and let the fanny muscles lower and lift your body. When sitting, don't let the weight of the body sink down on the hips so that your behind spreads out in the chair. Sit tall with the weight lifted and the buttock muscles pinched together. The derrière should not be the pedestal upon which the entire weight of the body rests.

Diet

Before you start to exercise, take a good look at yourself in a mirror. Check yourself in the nude, in a bathing suit, and in a tight pair of jeans. If you are broad in the beam, you probably need to lose weight as well as to exercise. Excess calories that are not used by the body are stored as *fat,* and lack of exercise contributes to overweight. But exercise alone will not burn up all of it. (In fact, if you are overweight and do body building-type exercises, you can turn the fat into hard bulk, which is extremely difficult to lose.) You may lose inches by exercising, but pounds can only be lost by dieting. Therefore a sensible diet is an aid to obtaining desired results from exercise. However, always consult your physician before embarking upon one. The fad or starvation diet can cause more harm than good.

Posture

While you are looking in the mirror, turn sideways. How are you standing?

• Are you pigeon-toed?

• Are your knees locked so that you feel pressure at the back of your knees?

• Are your knees thrust back (hyper-extended) so that your legs form the shape of a bow?

• Are you standing sway-backed with the lower back arched and your fanny sticking out?

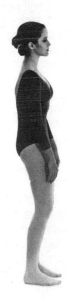

5

If the answer is "yes" to any of these questions, your bottom is going to look larger than it should. Bad posture emphasizes broadness and looseness. It contributes to bad muscle tone and reveals the flab that could be hidden by a better stance. You should stand with your feet straight ahead, your knees relaxed, never straight, and with your behind tucked under (see section on The Basic Pelvic Tuck), your back straight. Your appearance will improve immediately.

How to Exercise

The decision to exercise is not always an easy one to make, and is even harder to implement. Exercise can be fun and—especially when you know that you are actively doing something to better your appearance—it is also good for your morale. It will give you more energy, and your circulation will be better. Once you have been exercising regularly and can go at a fairly fast clip, your heart will benefit.

Start by picking a place where you can be comfortable. You may want to do your exercises in the privacy of your bedroom or living room. A number of the standing exercises can be done almost anywhere—the kitchen, bathroom, even the office. Make sure you have enough room so that your movements are unobstructed. When you do the floor exercises, put a heavy quilt or soft blanket on the floor. If the floor is carpeted, a sheet or soft bedspread should be put on it to prevent carpet burns.

Many of the easy standing exercises can be done in everyday clothes. For the others loose clothing, underwear, a nightgown, pajamas—or nothing at all—is acceptable. For fun, invest in a jazzy leotard.

For some of the standing exercises, you will need a support. A kitchen sink, a sturdy chair, a desk, even a file cabinet—anything that is approximately waist high and sturdy can be used. The support is for balance only. You should not lean the entire weight of your body on it.

Music is a great aid to the exerciser. It makes it more fun and sets a rhythm for you to follow. Although some of the exercises are based on yoga postures, others are modified from jazz and belly dance warm-ups and ballet barre movements. These, particularly, are easier if done to music. On several of these exercises, there are some suggestions as to the type of music that might fit best. Whether your taste runs to Bach or rock, pick what you like and let yourself go to the music. You'll feel great.

It is not unusual to hold your breath while exercising, especially if the exercises are new and you are concentrating. Try to overcome this quickly. It causes you to tire more quickly and is not beneficial. Don't worry about inhaling or exhaling at specific times while doing the movements. Keep your breathing normal.

In order to decide which exercises are best for you, it is important to classify the type of problems you have with your behind. First, measure it around the widest part. Be honest. Make sure you write down the measurement together with the date. You will want to consult this later. You may find one or more of these backside problems:

• The actual measurements are not so bad, but your backside is too soft and mushy to the touch.

• It sags.

• It is small and tight, but has crinkles under the cheeks.

• It is quite heavy and loose and saggy and crinkly.

• It is broad, fat, and muscular.

Determine what your problem is, then consult the section on "Classifying Your Rear" for which exercises to do.

To achieve the quickest results, you should exercise every day. If you must miss a day or two, pick up where you left off and keep going! Try to reserve some time every day when all the exercises can be done together, and when you are least likely to be disturbed. If that is not possible, try "sneaking" in exercises throughout the day, a few at a time. A number of the easier exercises are based on good posture and proper movement in everyday activity, and these can be done almost anywhere when you have a few spare minutes. Familiarize yourself with "your" exercises as quickly as possible so that you can immediately start making them a part of your daily routine. Read each exercise thoroughly *before* you start. Don't try to do them all at once. Begin with a few; learn them so that they can be done without consulting the book. Once you have mastered them, add a few more at a time. Always start the exercises slowly. Eventually, when you become proficient, you can do them at a faster speed.

Never jerk your movements. This can cause you to pull a muscle. Try always to move smoothly and fluidly whether exercising or in any normal motion. Don't overdo or force any movements. Work up to them slowly. Don't try to do all the suggested number of repetitions immediately. Even if you are an adept exerciser, you may want to do only half the suggested number in the beginning. Some people will be able to do more, and perhaps should. Unless you are an experienced exerciser in good condition, always start with the easier ones first, slowly progressing to the more difficult as you are able.

If you find that you are sore or your muscles seem to "burn" after exercising, then you are straining. Take a hot bath. Do a little less during the next session. If your muscles haven't been used, they will resist and complain when they are worked too hard. You must learn to listen to your body in order to know when you've had enough.

Bear in mind that just as every person is different, so is each body. Therefore there are some of you who will see a loss of inches and firming very quickly. Others will have to work longer to see the desired results. Don't become discouraged! Persevere! It is very difficult to see your own figure improve, as the change is gradual. A good gauge is in the fit of your clothes. Once you have made up your mind to start exercising, stay with it until you have obtained the desired results. Your moment of triumph will come when someone you haven't seen for a while comments on how great you look and how much weight you've lost, even though you may not have lost any!

Classifying Your Rear

Now's the time for the hard diagnosis. Which one of these is yours? Are you:

THE BRUTEOUS MAXIMUS
(broad, fat, and muscular)

This may be good for Arnold, but it is also the hardest to

remedy. First, you *must* go on a sensible diet. It is very hard to lose inches when the fat is hard and muscular. It can be done. It just takes longer. Reducing exercises predominate here, so you will need to concentrate on: "Hip Lift and Drop," "Let's Twist," "The Belly Dance Hip Circles," "Broadside Bump," "The Swivel," "Rump Ramble," "Swing High from Low," and "Swinging High." Of course, be aware of your posture and do the tucking and squeezing exercises. As you lose inches, start to add more exercises that firm and stretch, such as: "High Kicks," "Slow Blues Walk," "Bottoms Up," "Swinging Low," "Jazzy Swings," and "The Buttocks Lift."

THE CURDS AND WEIGH
(quite heavy and loose)

Inches come off a flabby body much more quickly. Your first goal is to lose some inches, then firm and tone. A diet is also a must. Reducing exercises again are predominant: "Hip Lift and Drop," "Let's Twist," "The Belly Dance Hip Circles," "Broadside Bump," "The Swivel," "Rump Ramble," "Swing High from Low," and "Swinging High." However, firming exercises can be added more quickly to your program: "High Kicks," "Bottoms Up," "Slow Blues Walk," "Swinging Low," "The Buttocks Lift," "Jazzy Swings," "Yoga Legs," and "Hipster." Make sure to always practice the pelvic tuck and squeeze both sitting and standing. You can immediately start to work slowly through the basic exercises. Leave the more advanced ones for a little later.

THE DANGLING DERRIÈRE
(small, does not need to lose inches, or if so, very few, but needs to remedy the jelly quality, sagging, or crinkly skin under buttocks)

Check your posture to make sure that you are standing correctly. Firming exercises are most important in your program. Practice all the pelvic tuck and squeeze exercises and start with the simple firming exercises, such as: "Slow Blues Walk," "Swinging Low," "The Buttocks Lift;" and intermediate ones, such as: "Butt Stretch," "High Kicks," "Swinging High," and "Strap Hanger's Stance." Gradually work up to the more advanced exercises: "Yoga Legs," "Hip Rotation," "The Doggie Leg Lift," "Jazzy Swings," "The Tangle," "Hipster," and "Leg Drag."

THE UN-BUN
(small, compact, firm, but needs some additional help for crinkly skin and some sagging)

You are probably already exercising and just shy of perfect, but need a bit more help. You are already aware of your posture and stand correctly. Since your program requires firming and stretching, you can go directly to the more advanced exercises, such as "Yoga Legs," "Swinging High," "Butt Stretch," "High Kicks," and most of all, "The Tangle," "Leg Drag," Hip Rotation," "Jazzy Swings," "The Doggie Leg Lift," and "Hipster." Always make sure that you are warmed up before you start. If by chance you are lucky enough to look this good without being in an exercise program, then you should start with some of the basic firming exercises before tackling the advanced ones.

Types of Exercises

While all prudent exercise is beneficial, certain ones are better than others in obtaining the desired results. Once you have evaluated yourself to determine the type of problem you have with your fanny, you will be able to pick the type of exercises you need to do. All motions of the body are complex. There is no exercise that stretches muscles without contracting others. Therefore since movements done to spot reduce will stretch and contract several muscles, a number of the exercises in this book will fit into more than one of the following categories.

Reducing Exercises

These exercises are effective in breaking down fatty tissue so it can be carried away by the bloodstream. Such exercises are not effective in an overall weight reduction program, but can achieve wonders if you want to lose inches in a particular spot.

Firming Exercises

When muscles are not worked sufficiently, they become loose and flabby. This gives the muscles a puffy and shapeless appearance. Firming exercises work these muscles, cause them to become more taut, thus supporting the surrounding flesh so that it looks firmer.

Stretching Exercises

For a great variety of reasons, but more often due to tension and bad posture, muscles tend to become bunched up and tight. This restricts movement and very often is the cause of aches and pains. Stretching exercises are those designed to lengthen the muscle fibers and reduce the bulkiness caused when the muscles are constricted.

THE BASIC PELVIC TUCK

For proper body alignment and posture, the pelvic tuck is essential. Look at yourself in a mirror sideways. Can an imaginary line be drawn from the back of your head to the back of your heels? Does your fanny jut out past the line? Does the small of your back touch the line or is there an empty space? If so, you are not standing with a "tuck," but are probably sway-backed and your stomach is protruding. Try to correct this by doing the following:

1. Lie on the floor on your back, your knees bent, your feet flat on the floor near your behind. Check to see if you can place your hand between the floor and the small of your back. If so, you are *not* in a tuck position. Try pushing the *small* of your back *flat* on the floor by sliding your spine downward into the floor while very slightly lifting hips upward. Keep your back there. If you can achieve this, you are in a tucked position. Get the feel. If you still cannot get your back flat on the floor, bring both of your knees toward your chest, holding them with both hands. As you pull your knees toward your chest, the small of the back will touch the floor. Keeping the small of your back on the floor, slowly lower one leg to the floor with the knee bent and the foot flat on the floor close to your behind, then the other leg. Don't forget, it is important to keep the small of your back "glued" to the floor throughout.

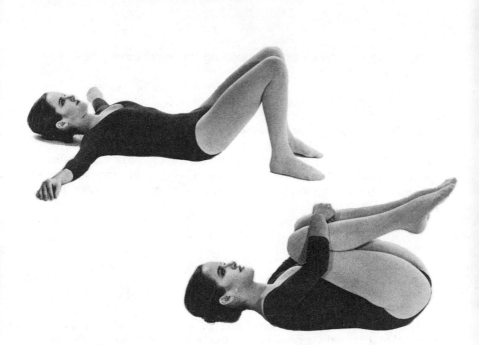

2. Once you have the feel of the pelvic tuck on the floor, try it standing with a support. Stand against the wall, your feet away from the wall with about a foot of space between them. Bend your knees just enough so that you can lean back against the wall in a semi-sitting position. Push your shoulders, the small of your back and your hips toward the wall until they touch. This will force your fanny to tuck. Your arms are close to your body with the palms touching the wall. Using your elbows and palms, push away until standing alone. Be careful as you push away from the wall that the position of your body doesn't change. You should try to remember how your body feels in this position and try to incorporate this "tuck" into your standing and walking postures.

3. Now that you have achieved the tuck both with the support of the floor and the wall, you are ready to solo. Stand, your feet separated about 8 inches. Place one hand on your behind, the other on your stomach. Bend your knees slightly so that they are relaxed and not locked or pushed back. With one hand gently push your bottom under and forward toward your stomach as you gently pull your stomach upward under your ribs with the other hand. Congratulations! You are at last standing with a tuck.

THE BASIC BUTTOCKS SQUEEZES

The Sunbather's Squeeze
Lie on your stomach, legs extended together on the floor, your head resting on your arms. Slowly squeeze the buttocks (gluteal) muscles together. Slowly release. Repeat 10 times and increase to 20 times. (For comfort and to lessen any strain on the back, you may want to put a small pillow under your stomach.)

The Pelvic Tuck Squeeze
Lie on your back, your knees bent, your heels flat on the floor near your behind. Slide your spine backward (tuck) until the small of the back is glued to the floor. Slowly squeeze the buttocks muscles together holding for 4 counts. Slowly release. Repeat 10 times.

The Standing Basic Buttocks Squeeze
Stand, your feet separated about 8 inches and your knees bent a little. Tuck fanny under (if you don't understand this, refer to section 3 of the Pelvic Tuck). Slowly squeeze the gluteals, holding for 4 counts. Slowly release. Repeat 10 times.

The Disco Squeeze Variation
Put on some disco music. Stand, as in the Standing Squeeze. Squeeze only the right buttock, lifting the right hip slightly. Drop the hip and release the squeeze. Repeat with the left. Go with the beat of the music for about 10 repetitions.

TIPS FOR SITTERS

When you're trapped sitting on an airplane, car, or bus, and especially at work, you can exercise your bottom. A few discreet movements will improve your circulation and muscle tone.

Sit straight, your feet flat on the floor, the small of your back * pushed against the back of the seat:

1. Practice the pelvic tuck. Push the small of the back firmly toward the back of the seat. Roll the buttocks under while pulling the stomach up under the ribs.

2. Holding the above position, squeeze the buttocks together. Hold 4 counts. Slowly release the squeeze. Do 10 times.

3. Roll the fanny side to side.

4. Lift the right buttock slightly up toward your right hip bone as the weight shifts toward the left buttock. Return to straight position. Repeat to the left. Do 5 sets.

HIP LIFT AND DROP

Stand with your feet separated about a foot, weight evenly distributed, arms at shoulder level or hands on hips. Keeping your upper body still, lift your right hip up toward your waist and to the side until your right heel comes off the floor, but keeping the ball of your right foot on the floor. Lower your hip into place and your heel to the floor. Do 5 repetitions on the right side, then 5 on the left. Do 2 sets. When you are adept at this, try doing 1 lift and drop on each side for a total of 10, using a quick staccato movement. Remember, don't arch your back and always pull your ribs and stomach up. This is fun if done to a quick foxtrot or Latin music.

LET'S TWIST

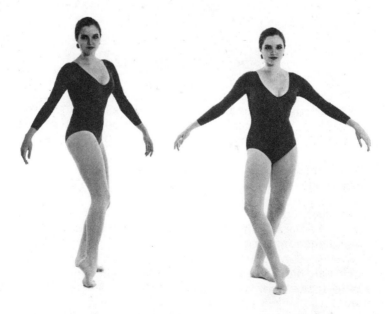

Stand with your feet separated about a foot, your right foot slightly forward with your weight resting on your left foot and the ball of your right foot. Rotate your right leg inward, with the heel off the floor, until your hip is high up and your toe and knee are turned inward. Rotate your leg outward, really "tucking" your right hip under and pushing your right heel forward as much as possible. Do 10 repetitions on the right, then 10 on the left. This exercise can be done slowly or fast. Put on some twist or disco music and try really twisting.

THE BELLY DANCE HIP CIRCLES

Stand with your feet separated about a foot, with your knees bent a little, arms at shoulder level or hands on hips. Slowly roll your hips to the right side. Push back on your fanny and roll your hips to the back (here, the back will arch *slightly*). Roll your hips to the left, starting to tuck your bottom. Roll your hips to the front with a quick pelvic tuck motion. Repeat, starting to the left. Do 3 repetitions each direction. Keep movements smooth. (Don't do this exercise if you have a bad back.) Try doing to Turkish, Greek, or burlesque music.

STRAP HANGER'S STANCE

Don't just let it hang there, use it! Many of us spend a great deal of time riding buses, subways, or trains. This is a good time to do the basic squeeze exercise with a little embellishment. The body flows with the motion of the vehicle as it slows down, stops, starts up, and turns corners.

Stand feet straight ahead and apart so that your balance is evenly distributed.

1. Bend the knees slightly. Tuck your fanny in. Slowly squeeze buttocks. Hold for 4 counts. Slowly release squeeze. Rest. Repeat as bus moves.

2. As bus starts to brake, rock toward leg in the direction of the front of the bus until the weight is on that leg, squeezing the buttock on that leg only. Have the feeling that you are helping the bus to brake. Remain in this position as long as the bus is stopped.

3. When the bus starts up, release that buttock and slowly rock toward the leg in the direction of the back of the bus, squeezing that buttock. As the speed of the bus becomes steady, come back to position 1 until bus starts to brake or slow down. Then repeat 2. Remember to keep both knees slightly bent and the bottom tucked under throughout.

4. As the bus starts to turn a sharp corner, one often gets the feeling that the bus will tilt over completely. Get in the habit of leaning in the opposite direction to the tilt of the bus. Have the feeling that by the position of your body you are keeping the bus from turning over. If you lean forward, tighten the backs of the thighs and the buttocks for balance; if backward, thrust the fanny under even more, putting the weight more on the knees and front of the thighs and tightening the fanny. Never arch the back. Keep it straight.

BROADSIDE BUMP

Stand against the wall, the side of your right "cheek" touching the wall. Gently bounce your hip against the wall 4 times. Turn slightly until the back of your right cheek touches the wall. Bounce it 4 times. Continue with the back of your left cheek, then the side of your left cheek. Then start with the left. Keep a rhythm going, but don't bump too hard. You want to gently break down the fatty deposits, not bruise yourself. Do this whenever there is a convenient wall.

SLOW BLUES WALK

If you are a beginner, you should use a chair for support in this exercise. Stand with the feet separated about a foot.

1. Slowly bend and straighten your knees in an easy bounce, 4 times. Keep your fanny tucked. As you bend slightly, squeeze the buttocks.

2. With your weight on your left leg, rise up on the ball of your left foot, extending your right leg in front of you off the floor. You should feel the buttocks tighten.

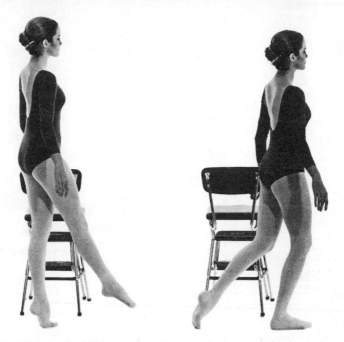

3. *Fall* forward shifting the weight onto your right foot, bending your right knee a little. You should feel the buttocks relax. Repeat the whole sequence now, starting with the weight on the right leg. Continue "walking" forward in this manner. Make sure that the feet follow one another in a straight line. This takes practice. Put on some slow "blues" music. It makes it easier and more fun to do.

⅄ SWINGING HIGH

The back of a sturdy chair, a sink, even a desk or a filing cabinet, provided it is approximately waist high and stable, can be used as a support.
Stand, sideways to a support with your left hand resting on it, your right hand on your right hip or at shoulder level, your feet together. Keep a "tuck" throughout this exercise. Swing your right leg up and forward. Swing your leg back and up. Continue a loose, easy swing, front and back, 5 times. Turn around and repeat with your left leg, 5 times. Always swing as high as possible without strain. Don't arch your back. Keep your stomach pulled up. If desired, repeat the entire exercise 1 or 2 more sets. As you become more advanced and can control your back, try

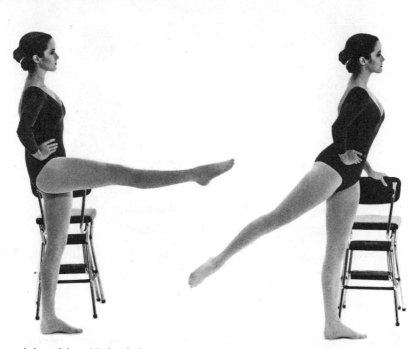

doing this with both legs turned out from the hip so that your feet make a wide V, or if possible, a straight line on the floor. Don't put any weight on the inside of your foot. Keep it on the *outside*. If you are using this exercise to reduce, keep the foot relaxed. If you want to use it as a firming exercise, point the toe of the working foot.

SWINGING LOW

Keep your upper back straight throughout this exercise. Don't arch. Kneel on the floor. Hold onto a support such as a bed, a small table, or a chair. Lift your right knee up toward your chest as high as possible. Swing your knee back through the original position without stopping and up in back slightly, your knee toward the floor, your foot toward the ceiling. Do 14 easy swings with the right, then 14 with the left. Don't go too fast.

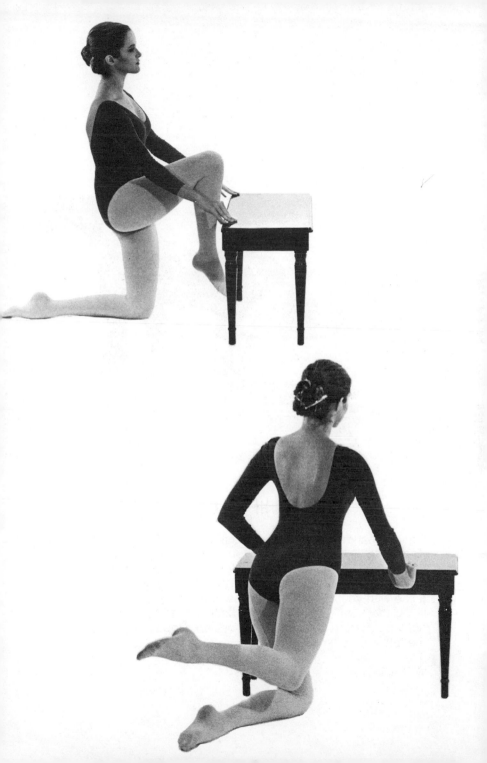

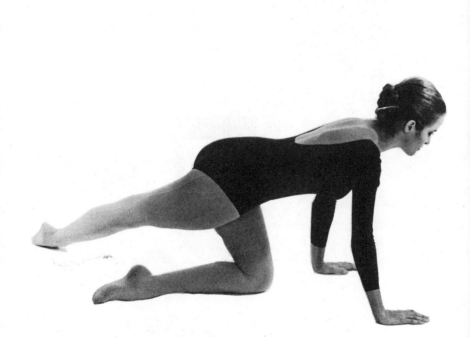

HIPSTER

On your hands and knees on the floor. Try not to arch your back. Keep it flat like a table. Cross your right leg behind your left. Your right leg is extended and your foot is flexed. Keeping your leg crossed and your foot flexed, lift your right leg off the floor until on a line with your behind. Try to feel that you are lifting your leg by lifting the heel. Lower it to the floor. Do 15 repetitions with the right leg. Return to the original position. Repeat the exercise with the left leg, 15 times.

THE RUMP RAMBLE

If you are generously endowed, try this time-honored favorite. Sit, your legs extended on the floor, your arms extended out from your shoulders. Take a "stroll" using the cheeks of your behind instead of your feet. Don't scoot. Pick up each cheek and put it down. Do 15 times. Now try walking to the side. Do 8 times to the right, 8 to the left. Do 2 sets. Repeat everything.

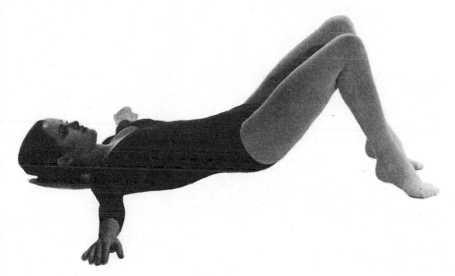

THE BUTTOCKS LIFT

Lie on your back, your knees bent, your feet flat on the floor near your behind. Slide your spine backward until the small of the back is on the floor. Lift your heels off the floor, keeping weight on the balls of your feet. Squeeze the gluteal muscles. Then slowly lift your behind off the floor keeping the tuck position. Don't raise your body any higher than your waist. Slowly lower your body to the floor. The small of your back must touch before your behind. Lower your heels to the floor. Relax your buttocks muscles. Do 3 repetitions.

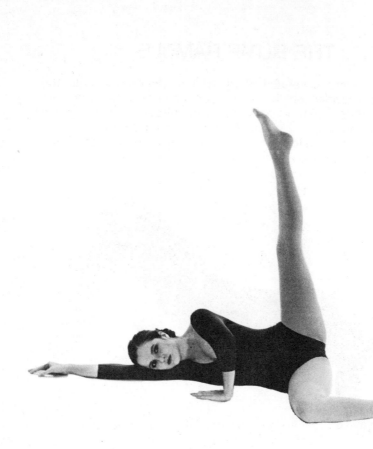

SWING HIGH FROM LOW

Lie on your right side, your head resting on your right arm, your left hand on the floor near your chest, your knees drawn up toward your chest in the fetal position. In one continuous movement, lift your top leg, keeping your leg bent until your knee is pointed toward the ceiling, and extend it upward. Again in one movement, lower your leg to the bent knee position, then back to the original position. Do 20 repetitions on the right side, then 20 on the left.

BUTT STRETCH

Lie on your right side, your head resting on your right arm, your left hand on the floor near your chest, your legs together and slightly forward. Lift your top leg slightly. Bend your knee to your chest. Keeping your knee in this position, push your leg forward directly in front of your chest, leading with the heel. Bend your leg back to your chest. Return your leg to the original position but don't lower your leg to the floor. Keep your leg off the floor throughout the exercise. Do 10 repetitions on the right side, then 10 on the left. If desired, repeat 10 times on each side.

YOGA LEGS

Lie on your stomach, your head resting on your folded arms, your legs extended on the floor. Lift your left leg off the floor as high as you can comfortably. Turn your leg out slightly from your hip. Squeeze your buttocks. Hold for the count of 10. Lower your leg to the floor. Repeat with the right leg. Repeat, alternating legs, 5 times each leg. Keep your hip bones and stomach on the floor, trying not to use the back.

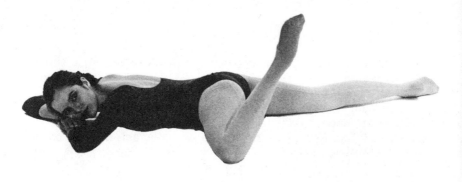

2

BOTTOMS UP

Lie on your stomach, your head resting on your folded arms, your legs extended on the floor. Stretch your left leg directly out from your hip, bending your leg downward at the knee. Your entire leg should touch the floor. Using your knee as a pivot, lift your calf and your foot off the floor until they are at a right angle to your knee and your thigh. Lower them to the floor. Lift and lower your foot and your calf 5 times before bringing your leg back to the original position. Repeat with the right. (If there is any pull felt in your lower back, place a small pillow under your stomach. Don't do this exercise if you have any knee problems.)

THE SWIVEL

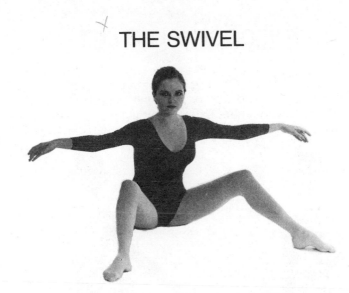

Sit, your legs open as wide as is comfortable, your arms stretched at shoulder level. Keep both your knees bent. Don't let your back arch or slump. Sit straight with your ribs lifted and your stomach pulled up. Rotate both your legs to the right until your knees touch the floor. Lift your knees up and rotate to the left until your knees touch the floor. Do 10 repetitions. (If you have bad knees, be careful of this one.)

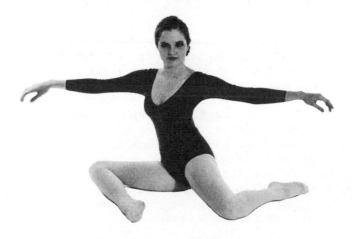

THE DOGGIE LEG LIFT

On your hands and knees on the floor. Try not to arch your back.
Keep it flat like a table. Point your right leg to the side. Lift your
leg off the floor on a line with your behind. Keeping your thigh at
this height, bend your knee. Extend your leg. Lower it to the floor.
Do 10 to 15 repetitions with the right leg, then 10 to 15 with the
left.

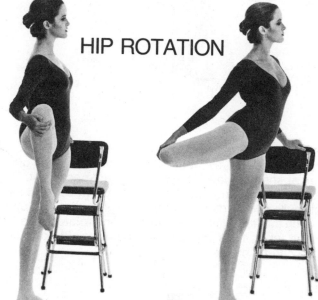

HIP ROTATION

Keep your back straight throughout. *Do not arch.* Stand with your
feet together, your left hand resting on a support. Lift your right
knee up toward your chest, holding your leg with your right hand
a few inches below your knee. Holding your leg throughout and
keeping your knee at this height, move your knee and thigh to the
side. Lift your hip slightly and move your knee and thigh to the
back. Your knee should now be at a right angle to your thigh.
Hold your leg in this position for 4 counts. Rotating your hip in the
socket, move your knee back to the side and again to the front.
Turn around and repeat on the other side. Do a total of 5
repetitions on each side. Make sure you are warmed up before
you do this exercise. It is a difficult one.

HIGH KICKS

Stand, your back toward a support with both your hands stretched back, holding onto the support. Your legs should be turned out from your hips to form a wide V, or, if possible, a straight line. Keep your back straight, your ribs lifted throughout. *Don't arch.* Kick your right leg off the floor toward your chest as high as possible. Return it to the original position. Do 3 more repetitions. Now, kick your right leg to the side as high as possible 4 times. Repeat entire exercise with the left leg. Repeat again with each leg. Make sure to keep both legs straight and turned out throughout the exercise. Keep the weight on the outside of your feet. If you are using this exercise to reduce your fanny, keep the foot of the working leg relaxed. To firm the behind, point the toe.

LEG DRAG

Lie on your back, your arms stretched out from your shoulders, your legs extended together on the floor.

1. Slide your right leg across your left until it extends at a right angle to your body. As you do this, keep pulling your right hip back from your leg in order to feel the stretch.

2. Pull your right hip back to the floor as you lift your leg above your body.

3. Lower your right leg to the right side toward your arm, keeping your left hip on the floor. Your right leg should be slightly off the floor.

4. Swing your right leg back to the original position. Repeat 8 times. Continue using your right leg, reversing the entire exercise: swinging your right leg out toward your right hand, lifting your leg up, crossing the body, sliding your leg back across the left to the original position. Do 8 repetitions with the left leg, then reverse the left 8 times.

JAZZY SWINGS

Throughout this exercise keep your back straight, *don't arch*. Keep your ribs lifted, your stomach pulled up, your bottom tucked, tightening the buttocks. Stand sideways to a support with your left hand resting on it, feet separated about 8 inches.

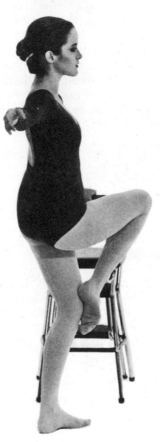

1. Rise up on the balls of your feet.

2. With your left heel on the floor, bend your left knee slightly while lifting your right knee up and across your body toward the left side.

3. Rise up on the ball of your left foot while rotating your right knee and thigh out toward the right side, in a continuous motion, extending your leg at the side as high as possible. Your toes are pointed toward the floor.

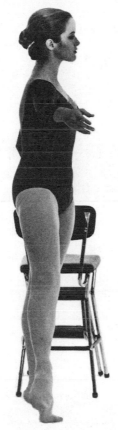

4. Place your right foot on the floor about a foot from the left. Your feet should be parallel and your toes straight ahead. Bend both your knees, tightening your buttocks as you bend.

Slide your right foot back to the original position and do a total of 8 repetitions. Then do 8 on the other side. Once you know the exercise, try doing it with fluid movements, counting 1 count for each part.

THE TANGLE

Lie on your back, your arms stretched straight out from your shoulders.

1. Bend your left knee with your foot on the floor near your bottom, your right leg extended on the floor.

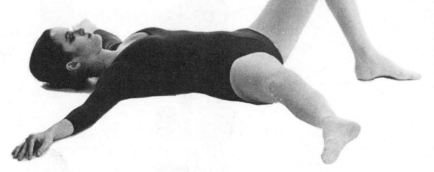

2. Swing your right leg—slightly off the floor—out to the side toward your right hand. Keep your behind on the floor.

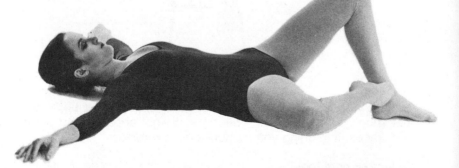

3. Your right thigh remains in this position while you bend your lower leg in toward your left leg, the toes touching the left ankle bone. Keep your behind on the floor.

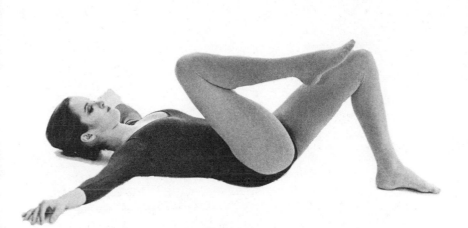

4. Keeping your knee bent, rotate your right leg and pull your knee close to your chest in one movement.

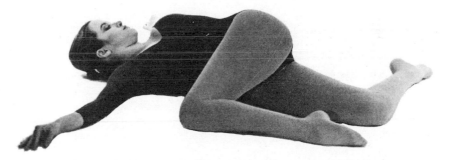

5. Rotate your right knee and hip across your body and left knee and hip until both knees touch the floor on the left side. Keep your shoulders on the floor.

Reverse the exercise. Do 5 to 10 repetitions with the right leg, then 5 to 10 with the left.

(If you have back problems, do not do this one because of the slight twisting involved.)

HELLSING ②

平野耕太
KOHTA HIRANO

translation
DUANE JOHNSON

lettering
WILBERT LACUNA

DARK HORSE MANGA

DMP
Digital Manga
Publishing

publishers
MIKE RICHARDSON and HIKARU SASAHARA

editors
TIM ERVIN-GORE and FRED LUI

collection designer
DAVID NESTELLE

English-language version produced by
DARK HORSE COMICS and DIGITAL MANGA PUBLISHING

HELLSING VOL.2

published by
Dark Horse Manga
a division of Dark Horse Comics, Inc.
10956 S.E. Main Street
Milwaukie, OR 97222

www.darkhorse.com

Digital Manga Publishing
1123 Dominguez Street, unit K
Carson, CA 90746

www.emanga.com

To find a comics shop in your area, call the
Comic Shop Locator Service toll-free at 1-888-266-4226

First edition: March 2004
ISBN: 1-59307-057-8

1 3 5 7 9 10 8 6 4 2

Printed in Canada

HELLSING ②

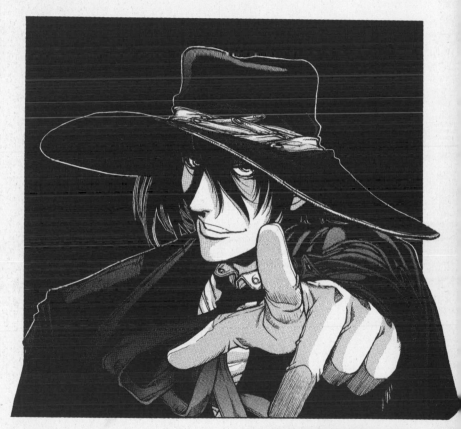

平野耕太

KOHTA HIRANO

HELLSING ②

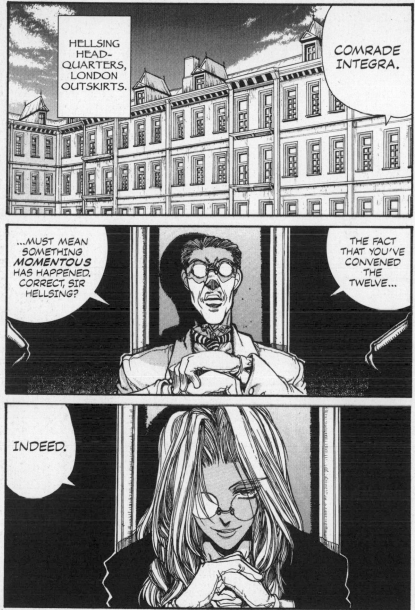

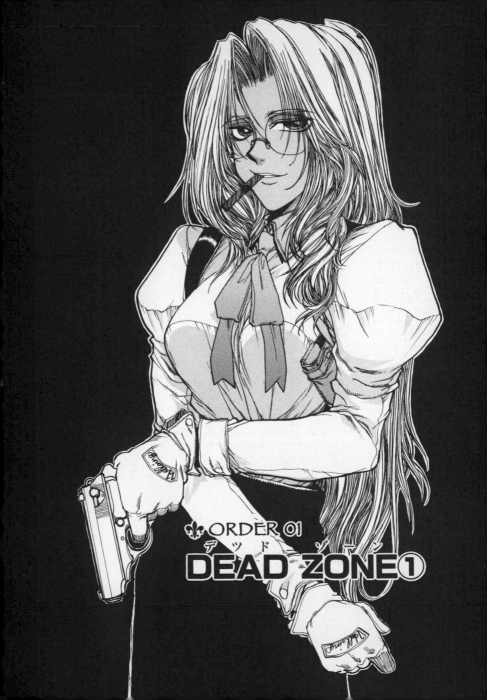

ORDER 01
DEAD ZONE①

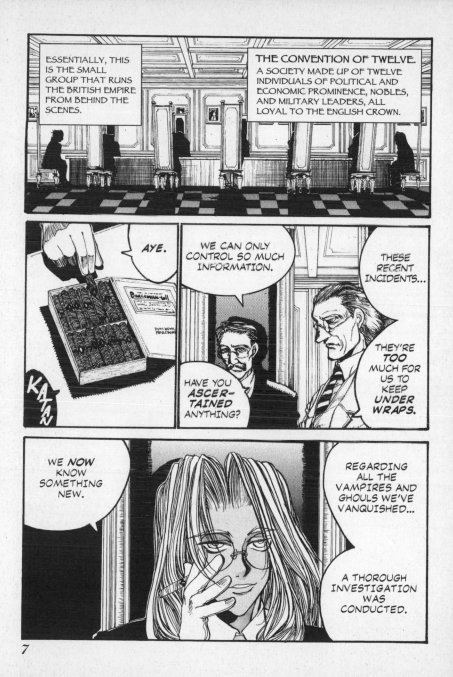

ESSENTIALLY, THIS IS THE SMALL GROUP THAT RUNS THE BRITISH EMPIRE FROM BEHIND THE SCENES.

THE CONVENTION OF TWELVE. A SOCIETY MADE UP OF TWELVE INDIVIDUALS OF POLITICAL AND ECONOMIC PROMINENCE, NOBLES, AND MILITARY LEADERS, ALL LOYAL TO THE ENGLISH CROWN.

AYE.

WE CAN ONLY CONTROL SO MUCH INFORMATION.

THESE RECENT INCIDENTS...

KATAN

HAVE YOU ASCER-TAINED ANYTHING?

THEY'RE TOO MUCH FOR US TO KEEP UNDER WRAPS.

WE NOW KNOW SOMETHING NEW.

REGARDING ALL THE VAMPIRES AND GHOULS WE'VE VANQUISHED...

A THOROUGH INVESTIGATION WAS CONDUCTED.

7

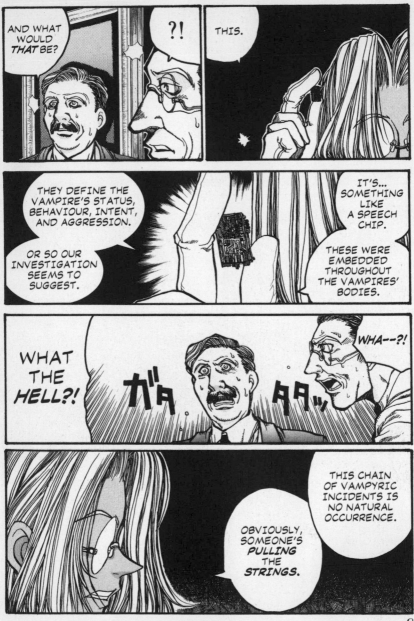

8

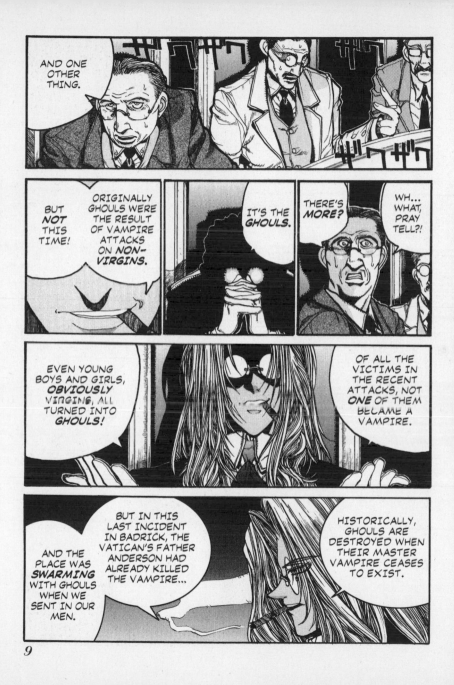

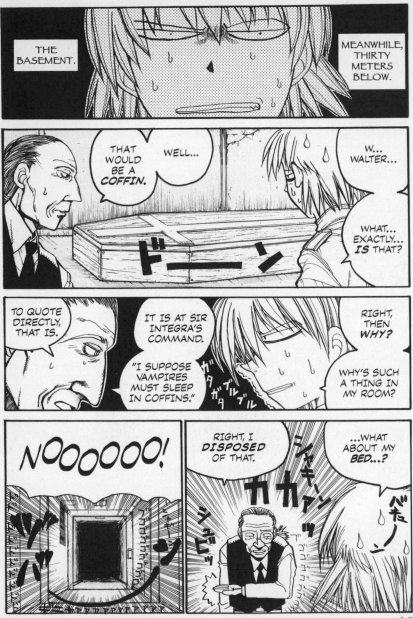

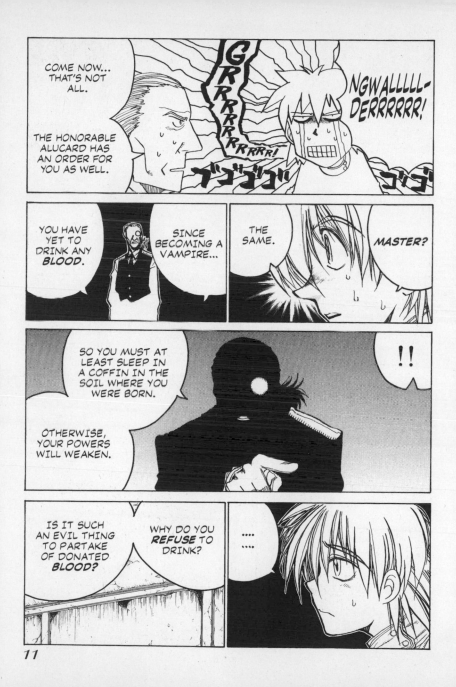

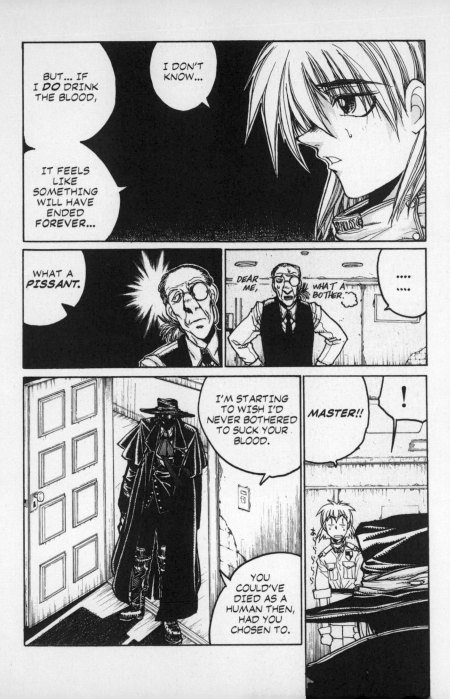

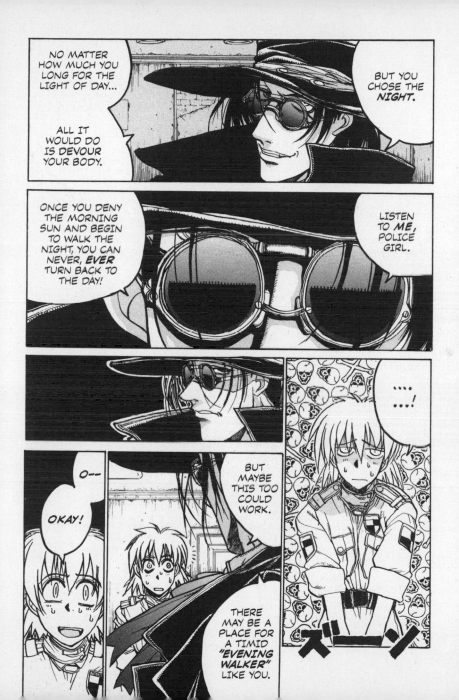

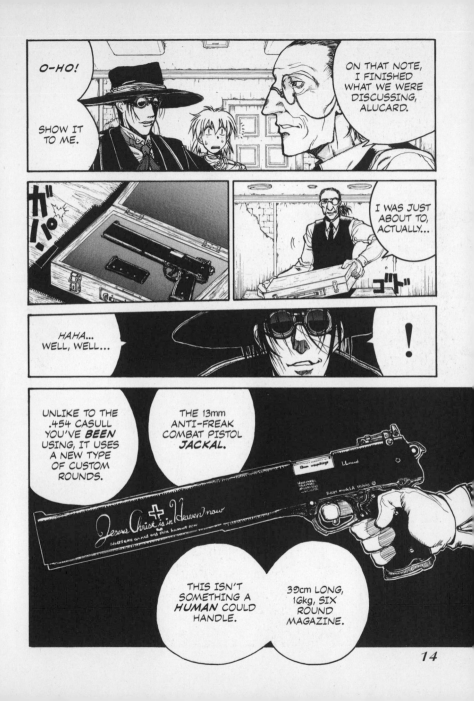

14

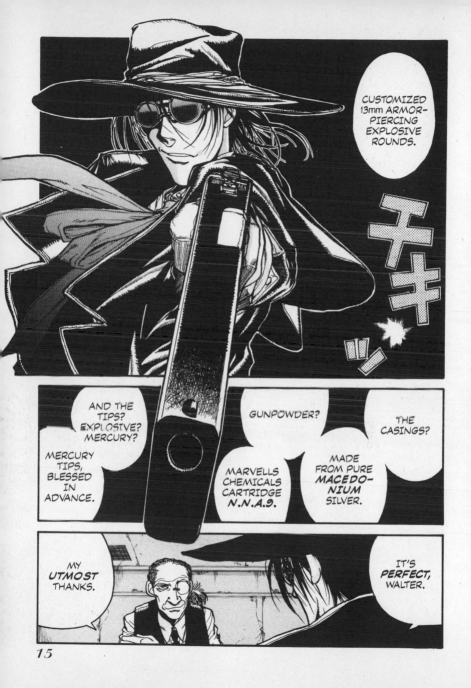

CUSTOMIZED 13mm ARMOR-PIERCING EXPLOSIVE ROUNDS.

AND THE TIPS? EXPLOSIVE? MERCURY?

MERCURY TIPS, BLESSED IN ADVANCE.

GUNPOWDER?

MARVELLS CHEMICALS CARTRIDGE *N.N.A.9.*

THE CASINGS?

MADE FROM PURE *MACEDO-NIUM* SILVER.

MY *UTMOST* THANKS.

IT'S *PERFECT,* WALTER.

15

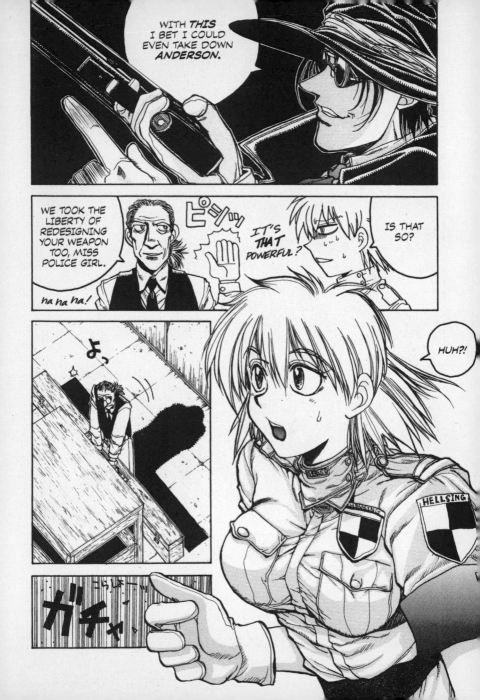

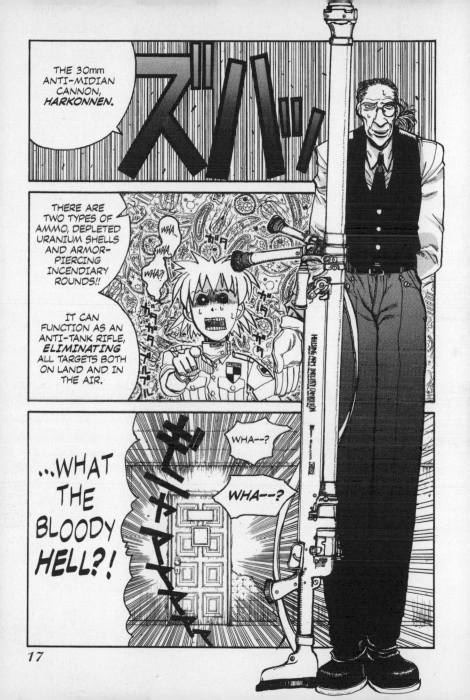

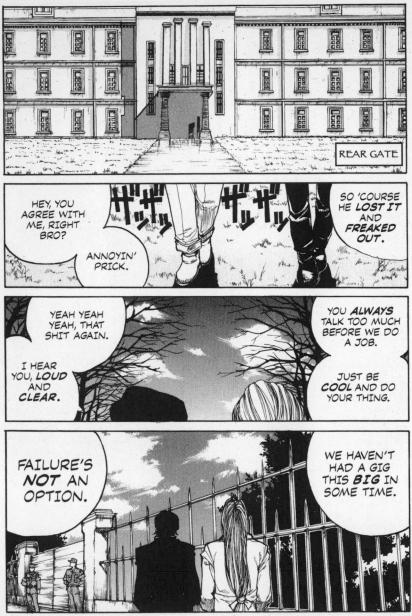

REAR GATE

18

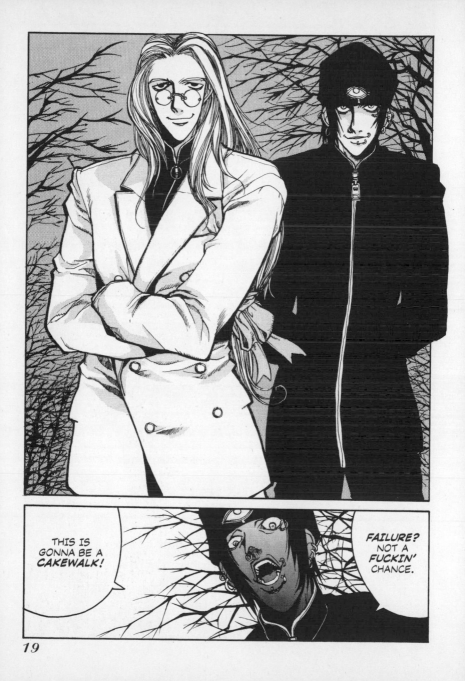

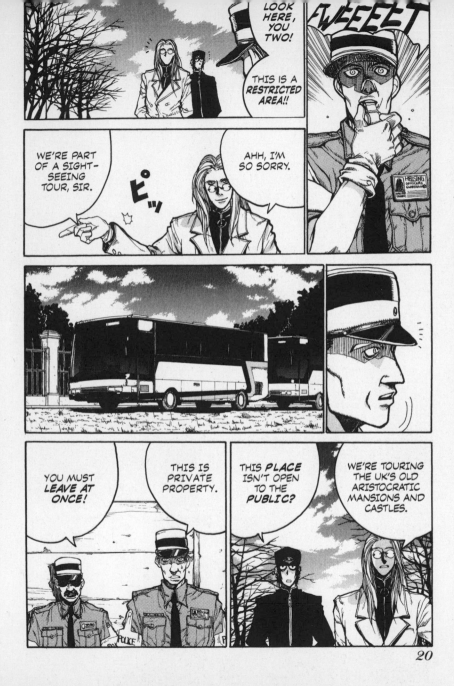

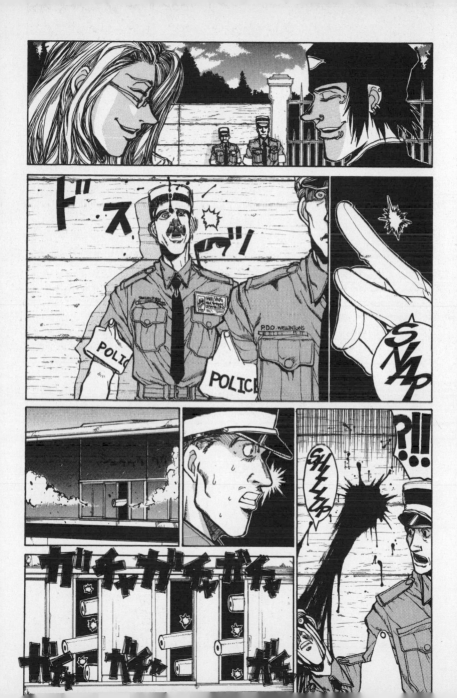

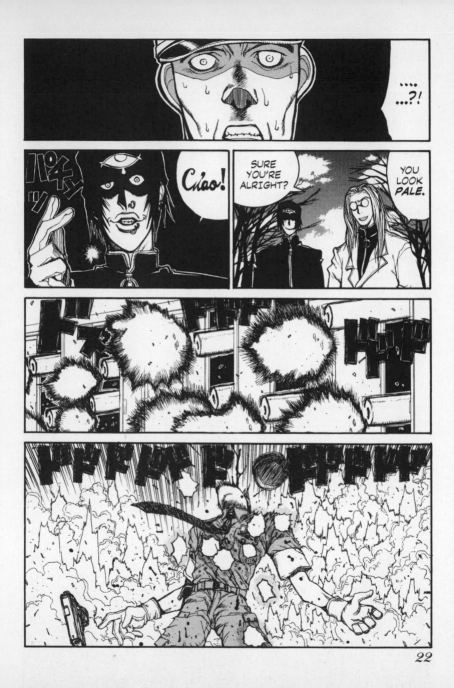

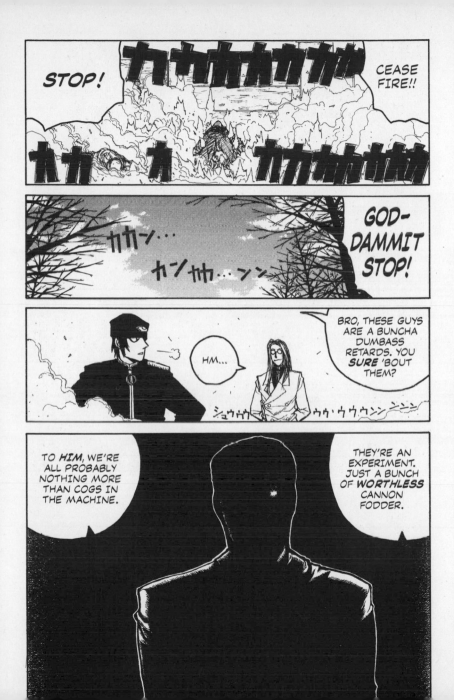

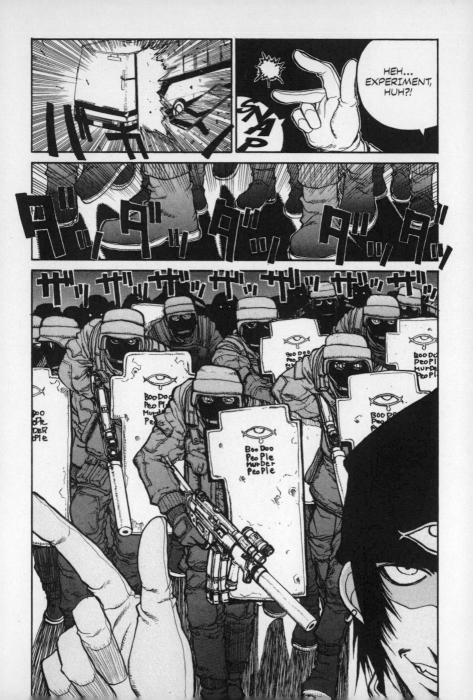

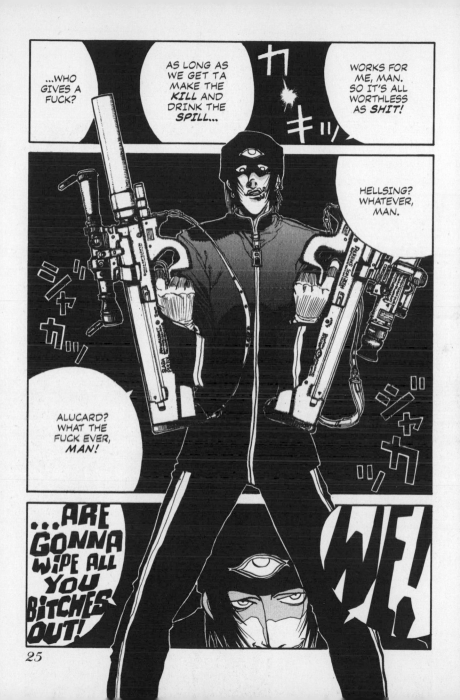

25

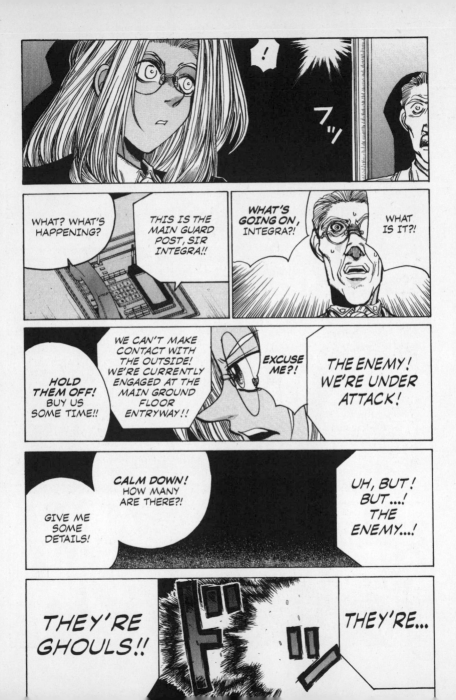

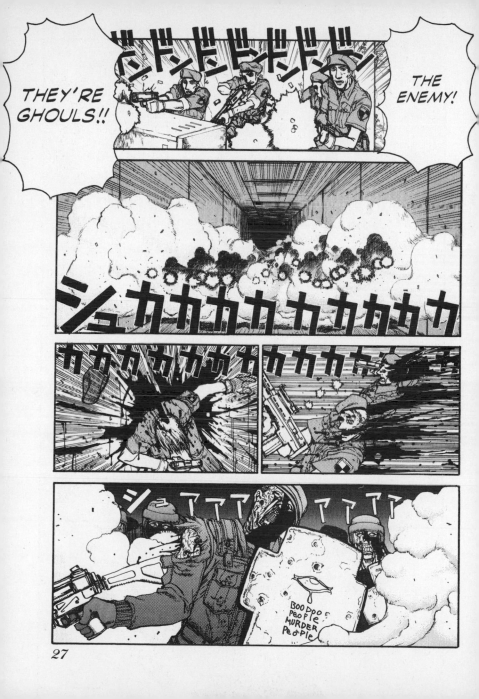

27

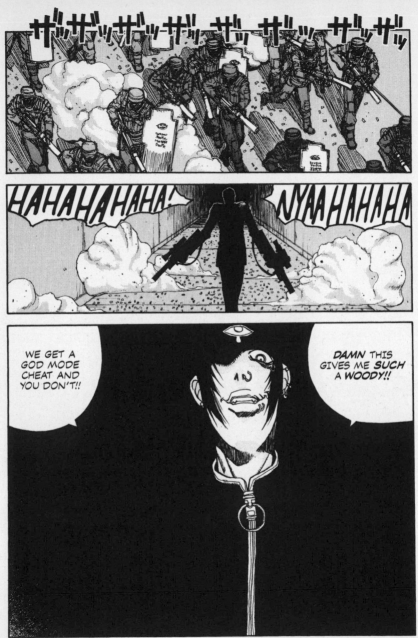

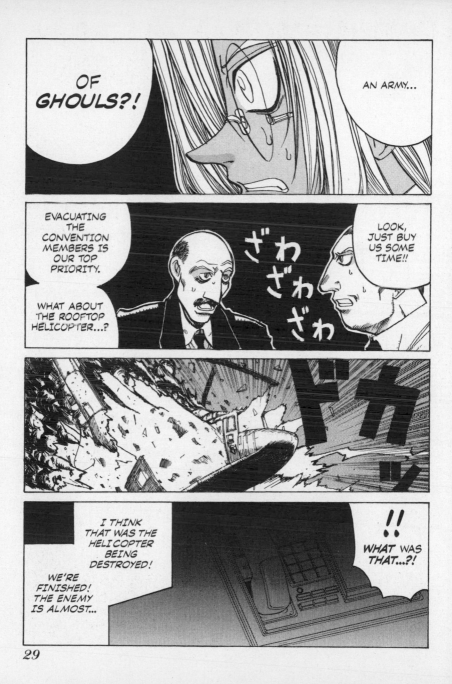

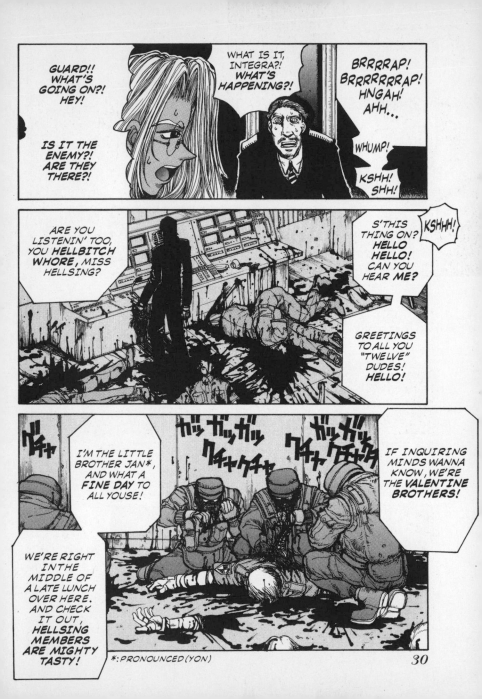

*:PRONOUNCED (YON)

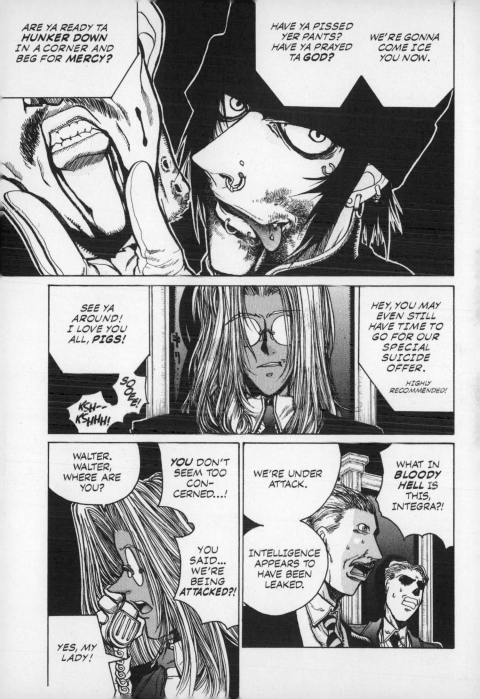

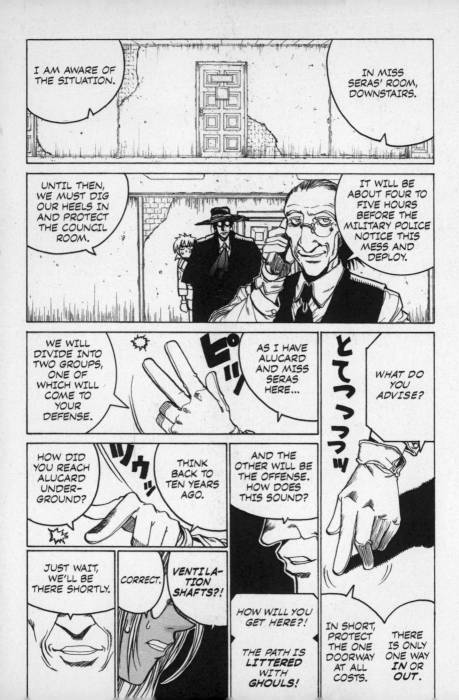

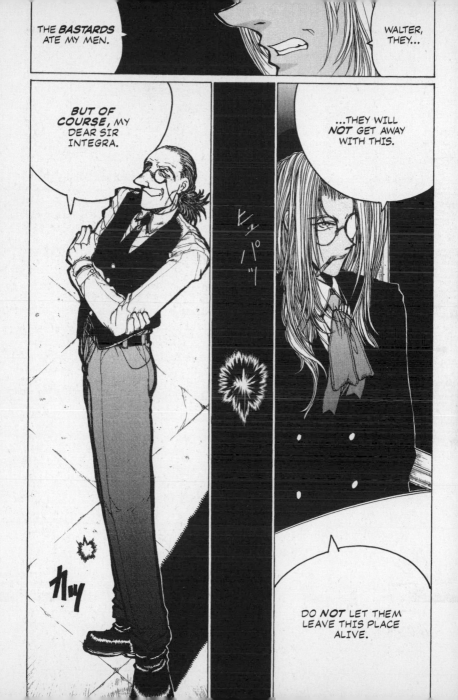

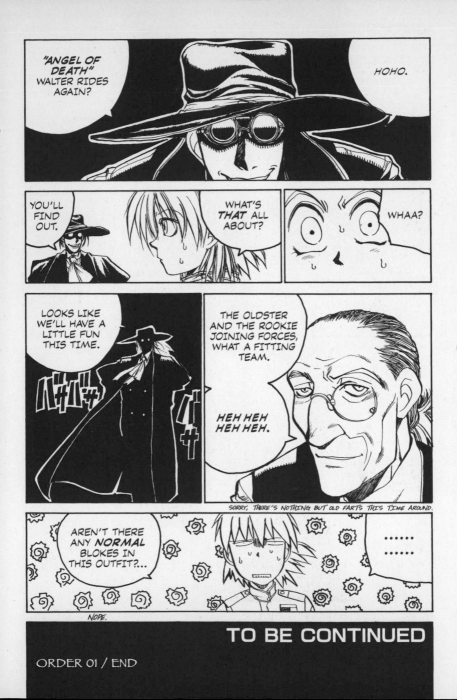

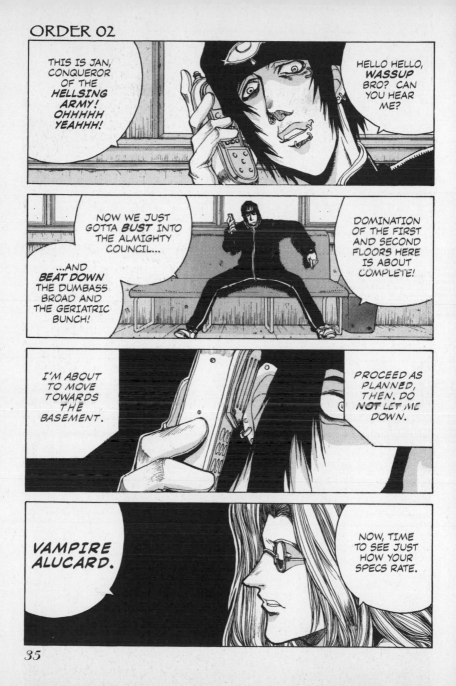

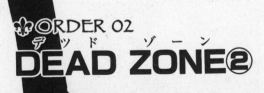

ORDER 02
DEAD ZONE②

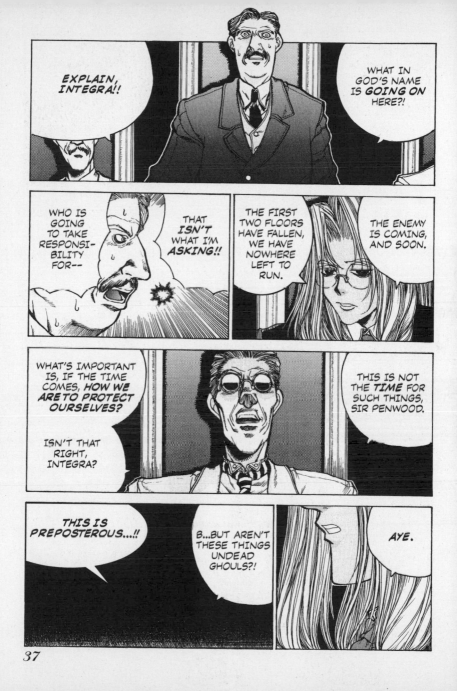

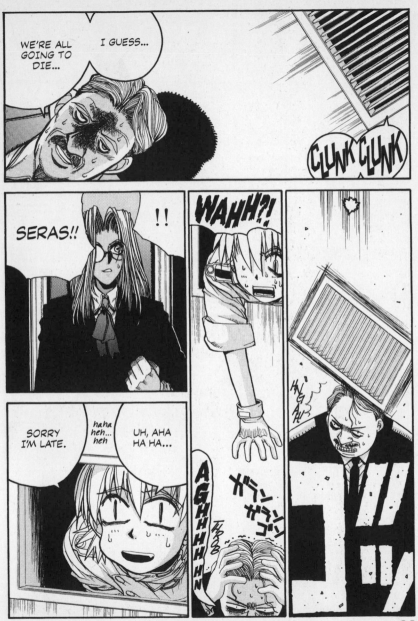

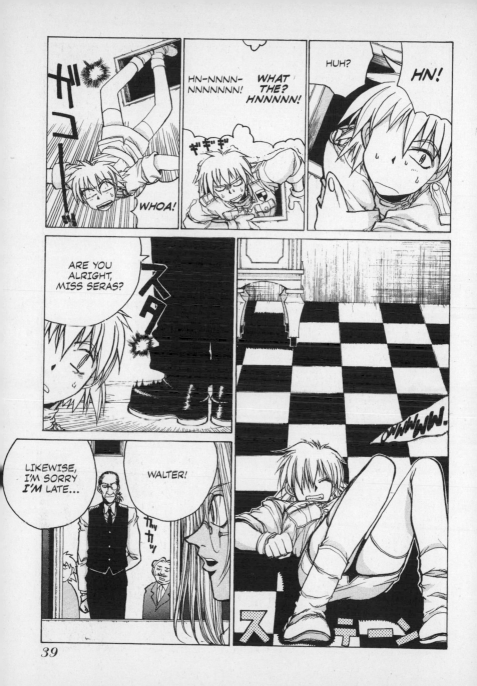

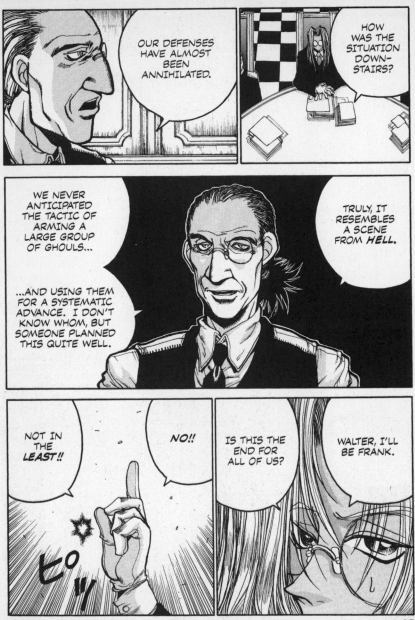

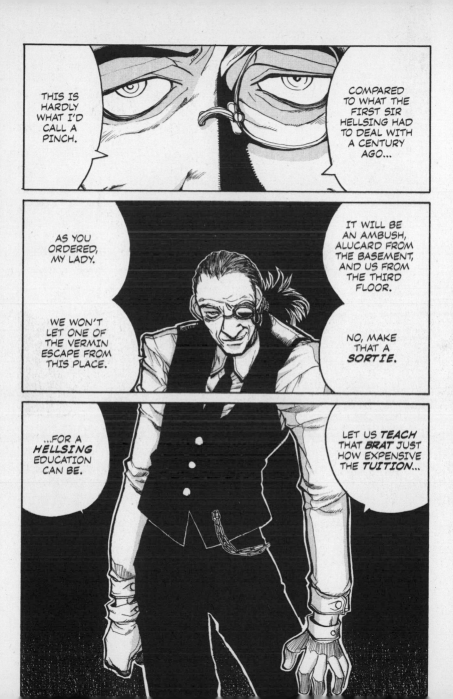

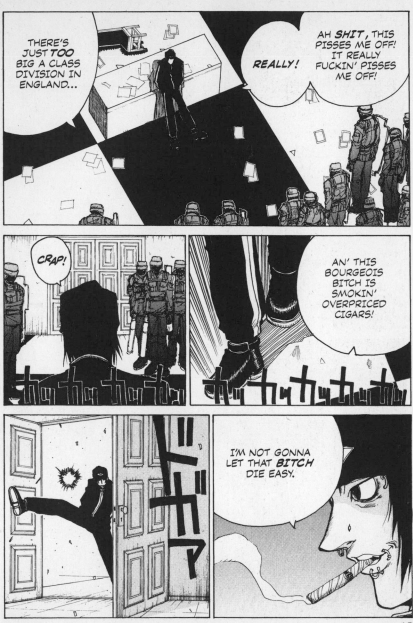

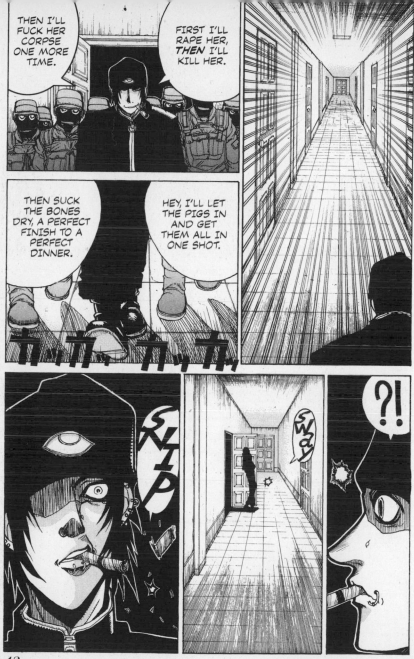

43

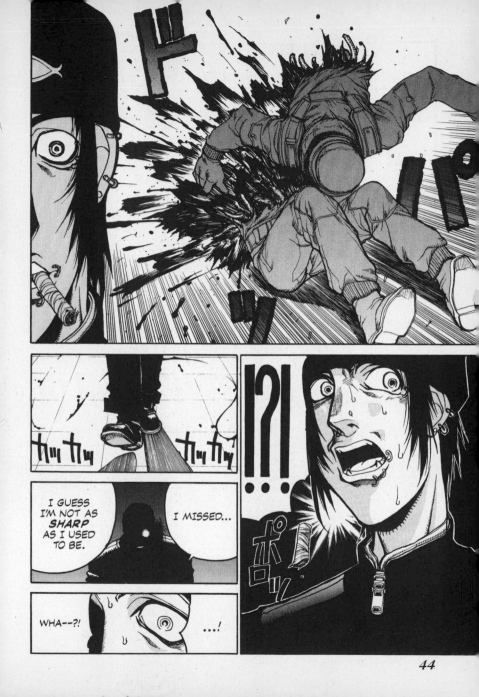

I GUESS I'M NOT AS *SHARP* AS I USED TO BE.

I MISSED...

WHA--?!

....!

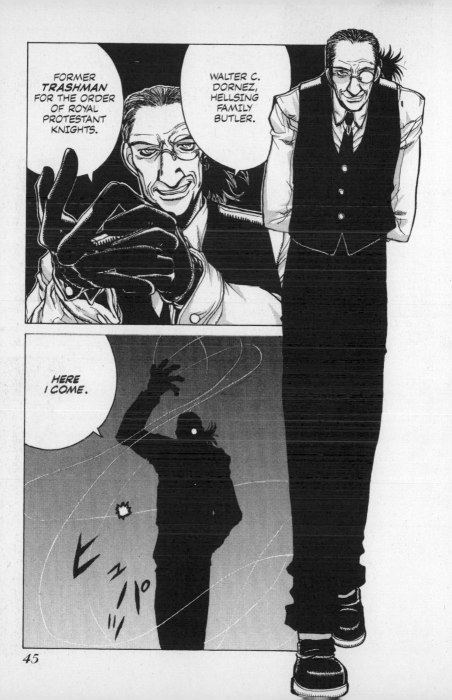

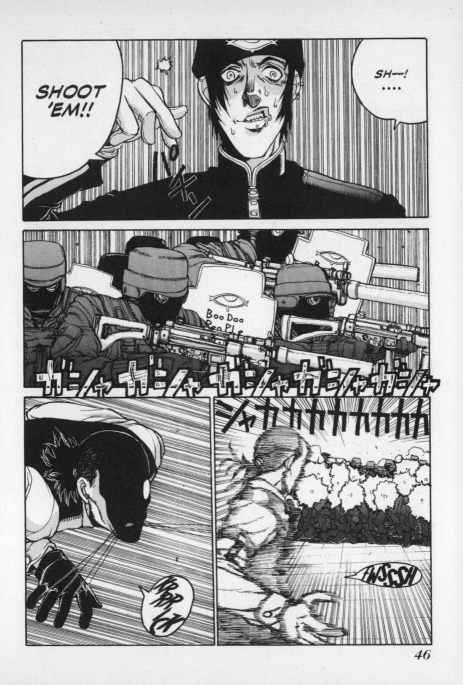

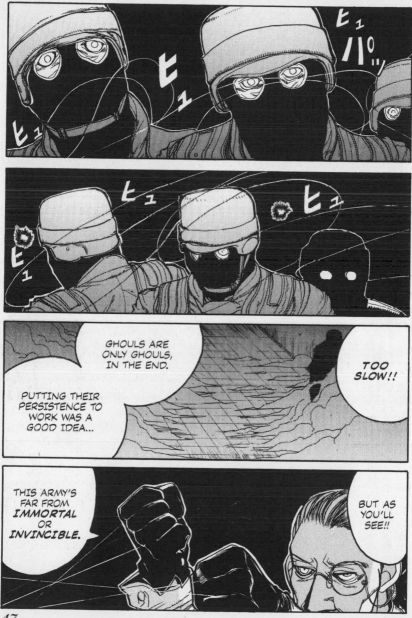

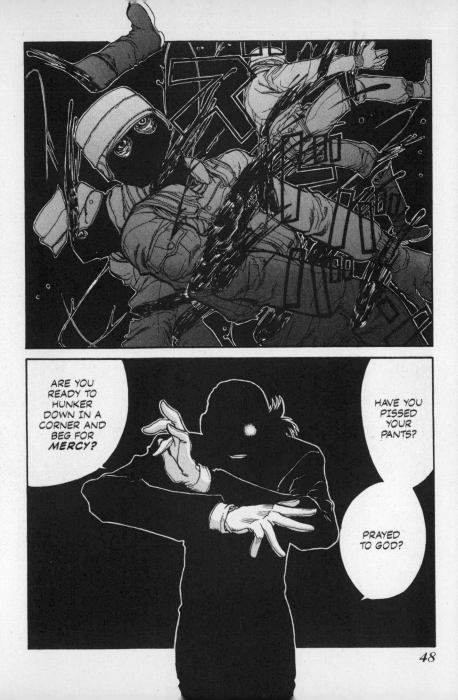

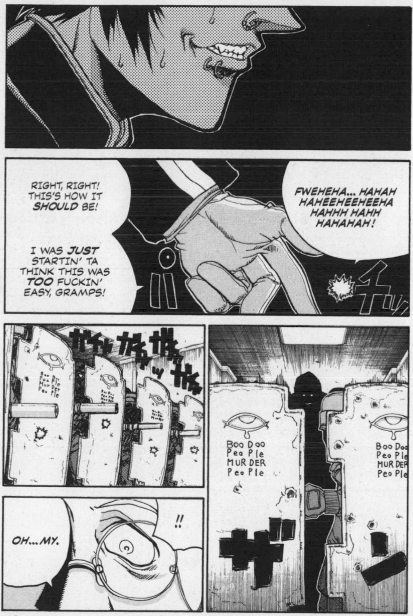

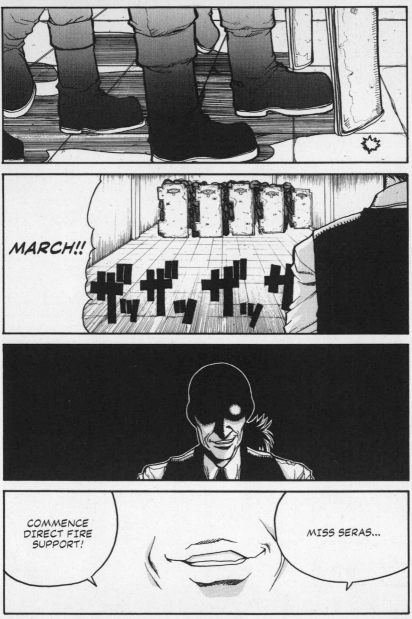

MARCH!!

COMMENCE
DIRECT FIRE
SUPPORT!

MISS SERAS...

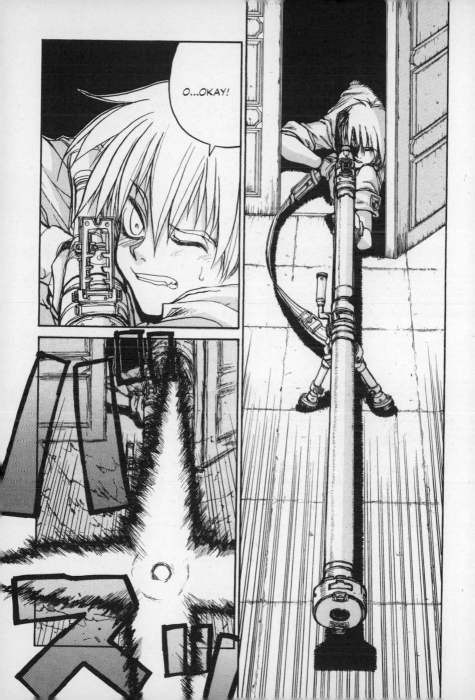

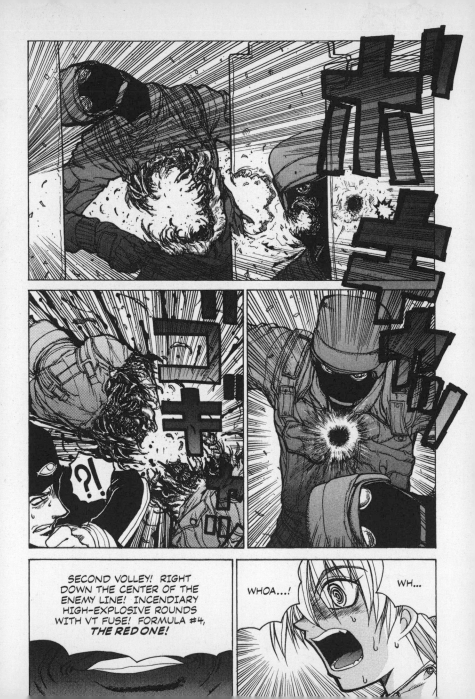

SECOND VOLLEY! RIGHT
DOWN THE CENTER OF THE
ENEMY LINE! INCENDIARY
HIGH-EXPLOSIVE ROUNDS
WITH VT FUSE! FORMULA #4,
THE RED ONE!

WHOA...!

WH...

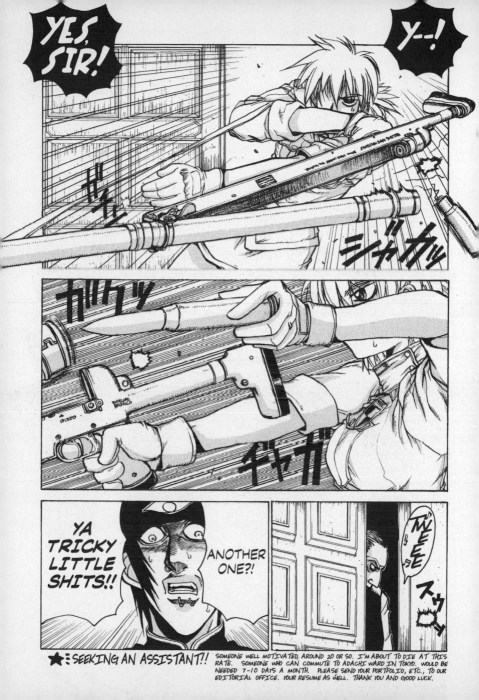

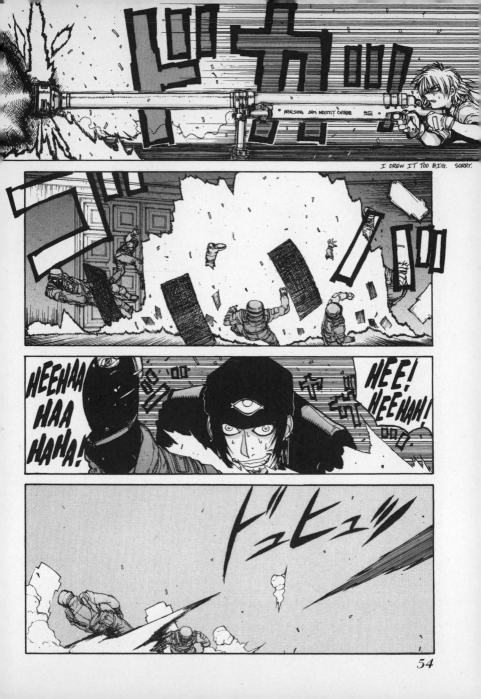

I DREW IT TOO BIG. SORRY.

54

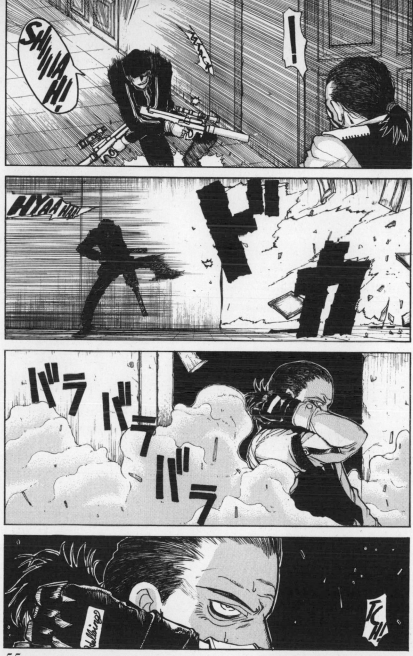

55

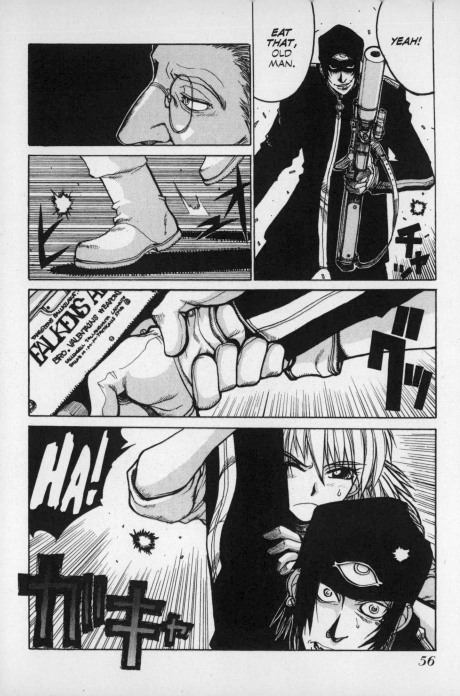

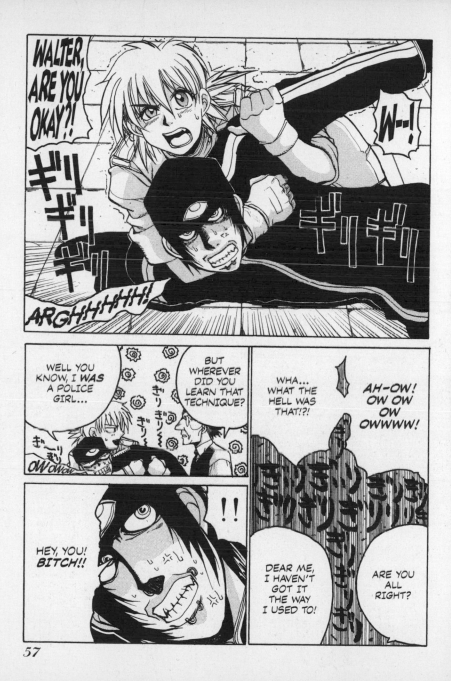

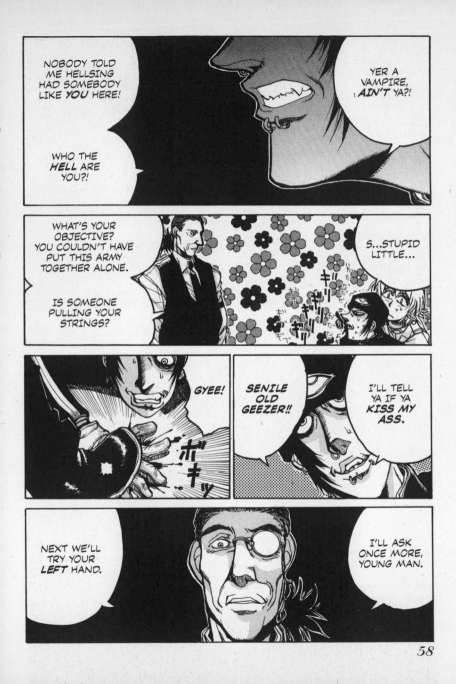

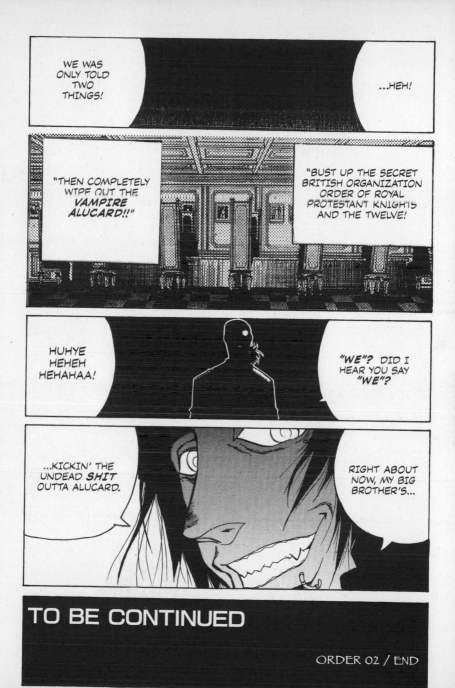

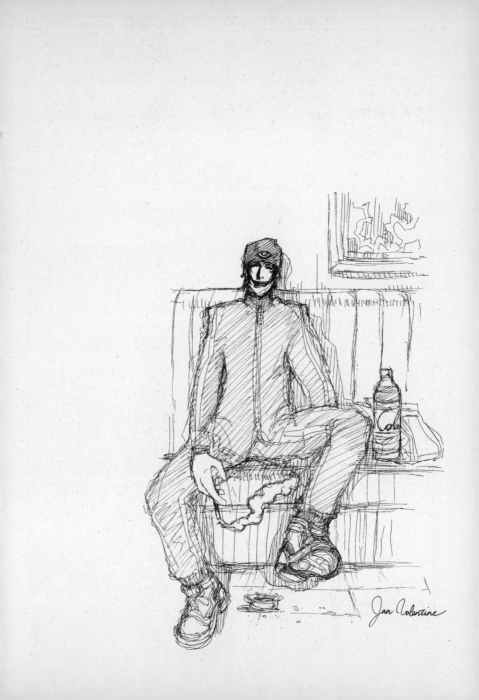

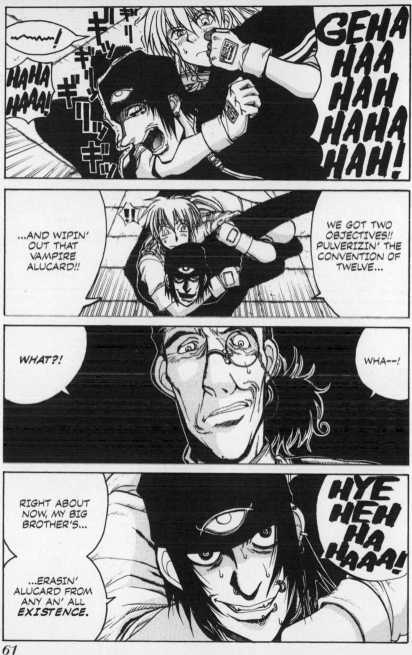

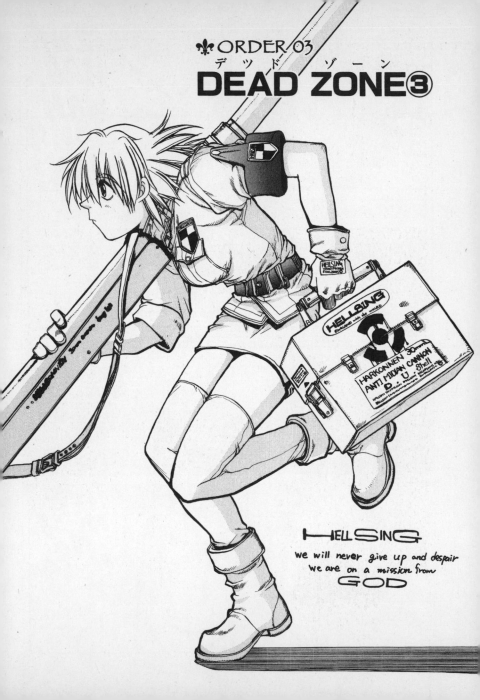

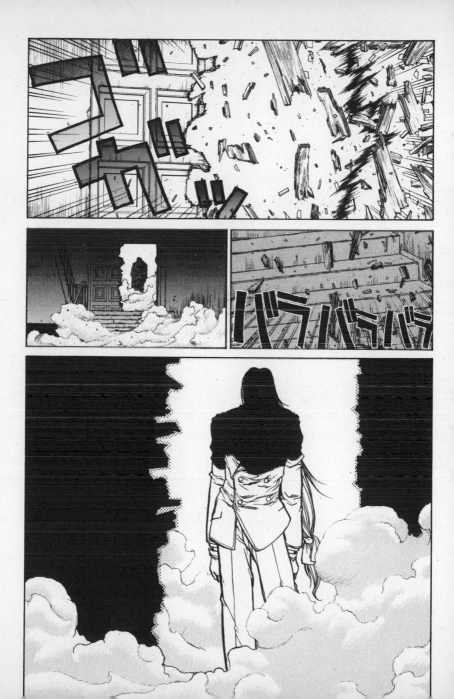

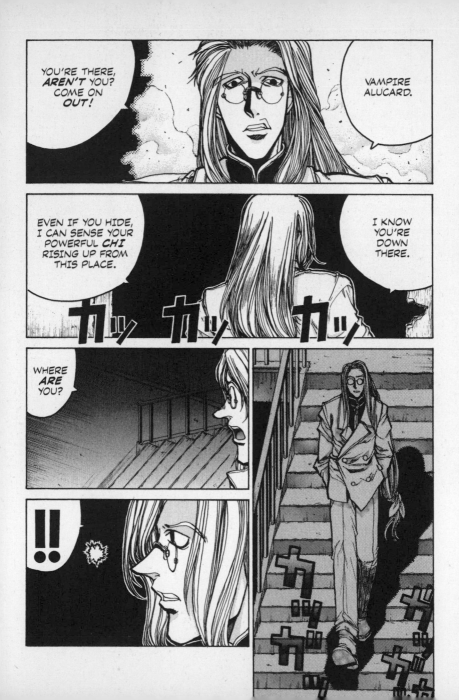

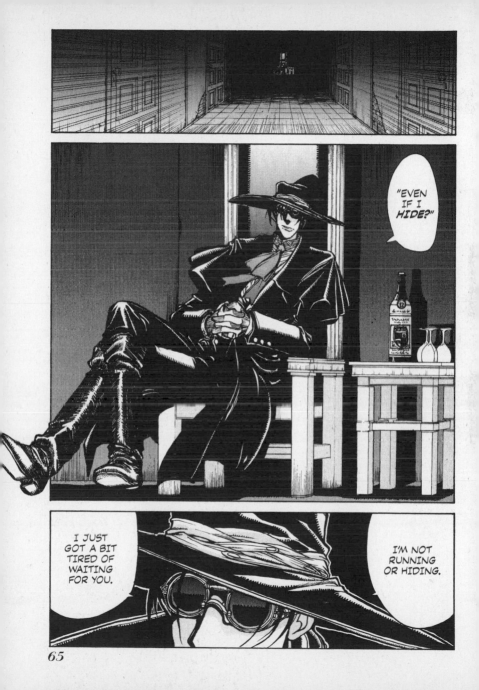

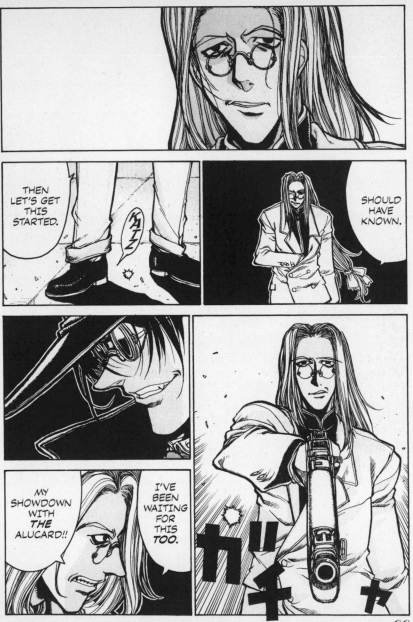

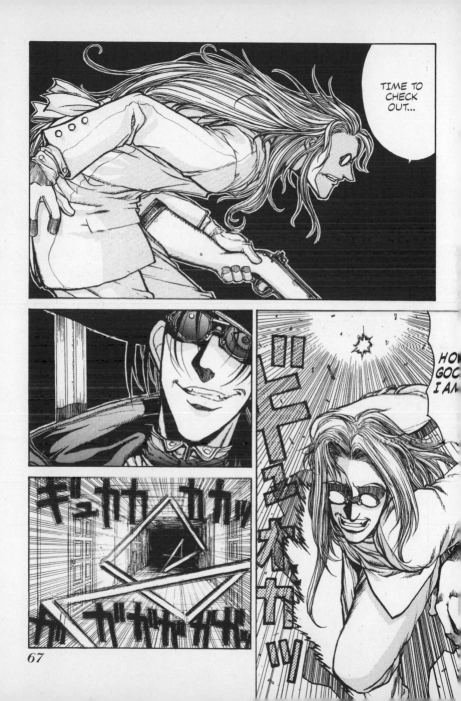

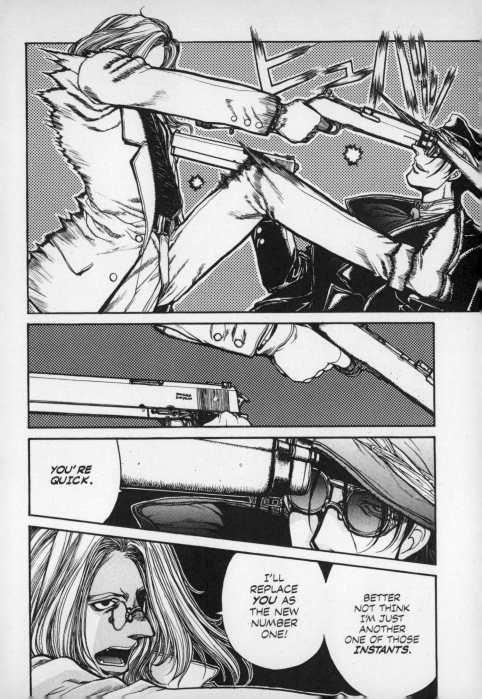

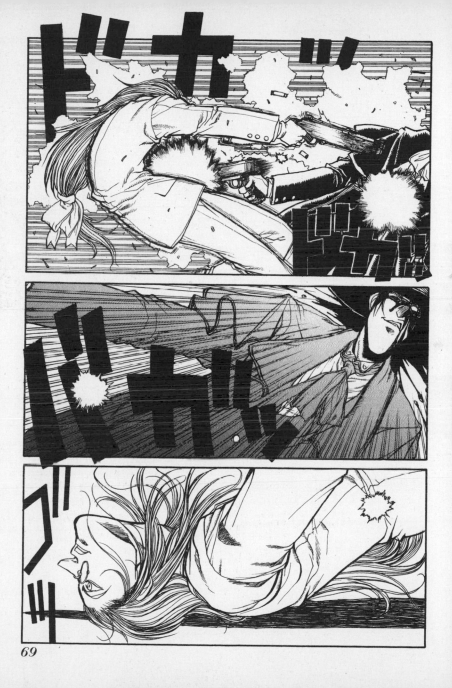

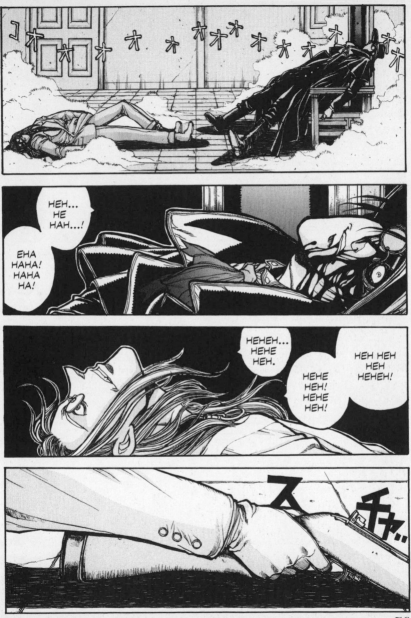

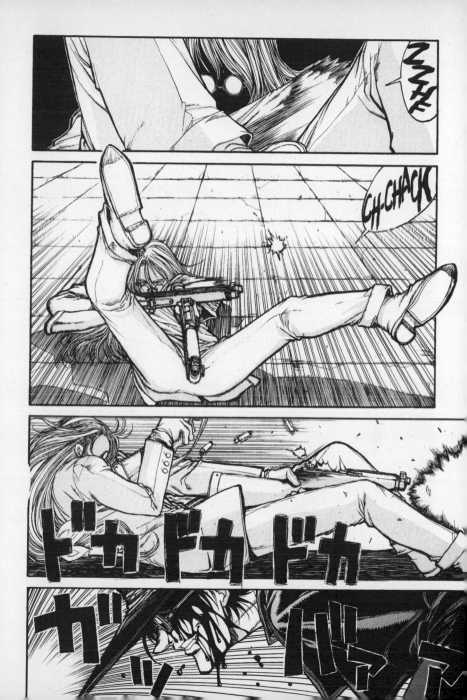

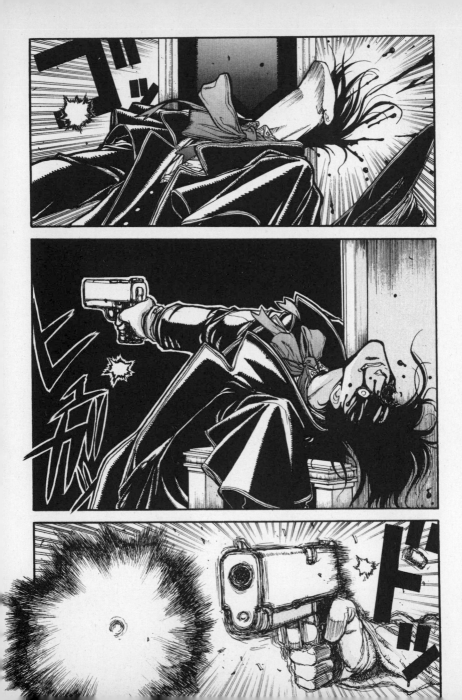

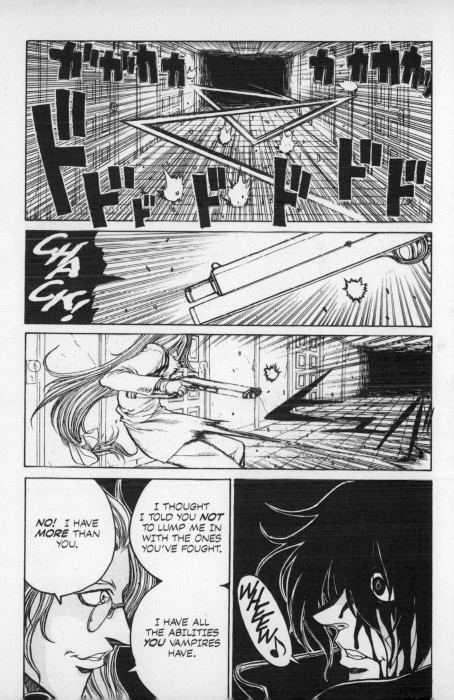

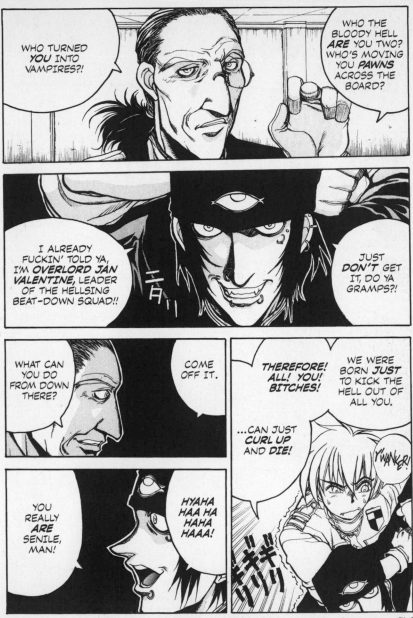

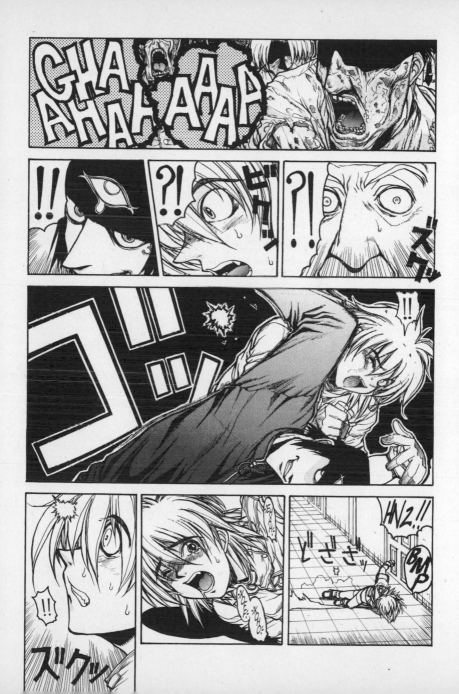

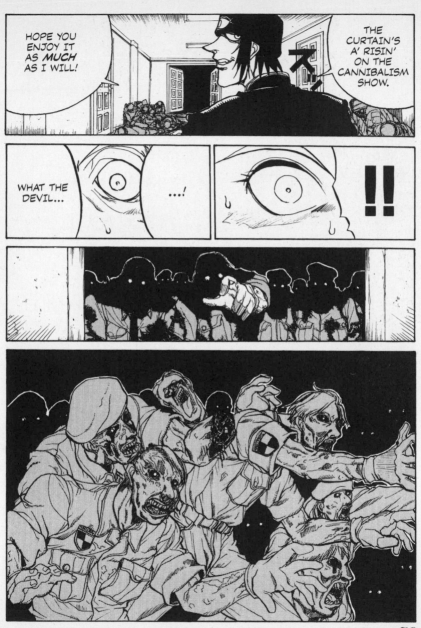

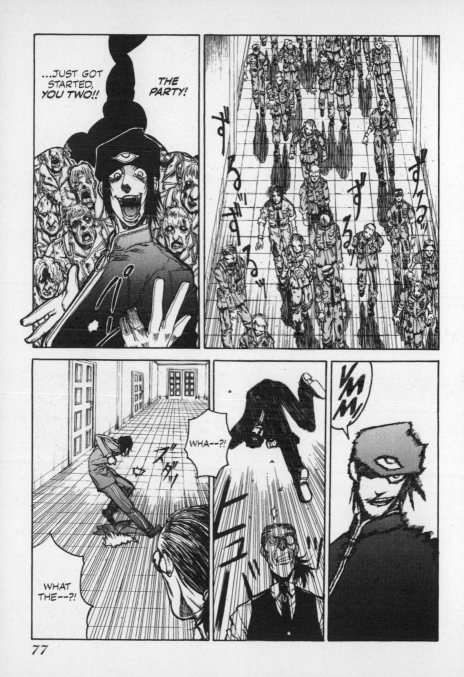

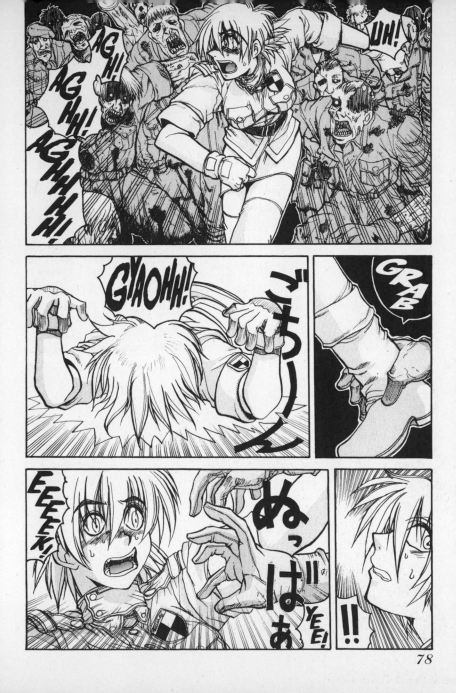

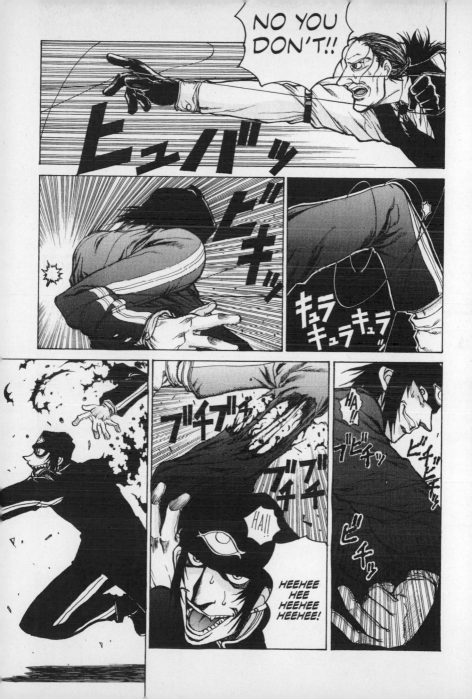

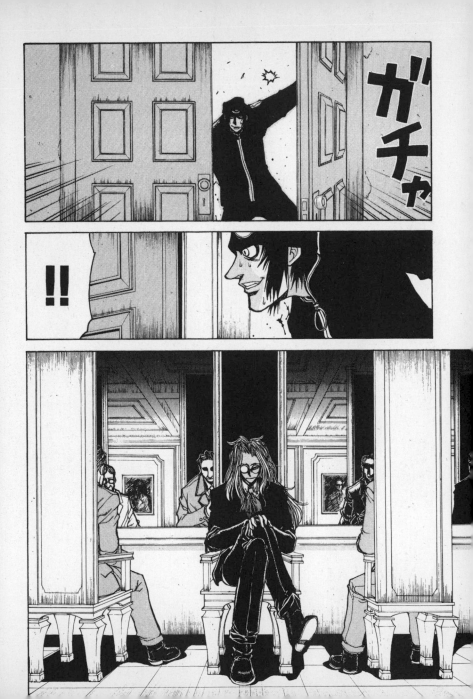

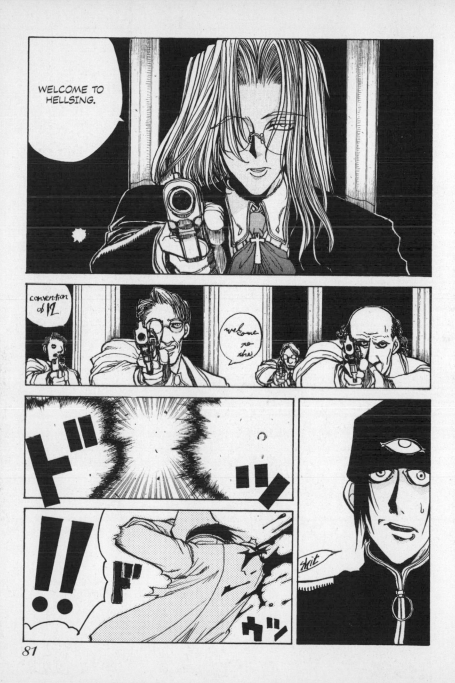

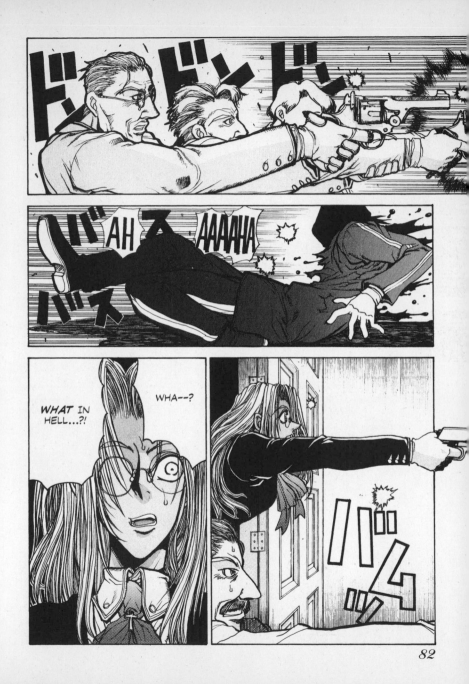

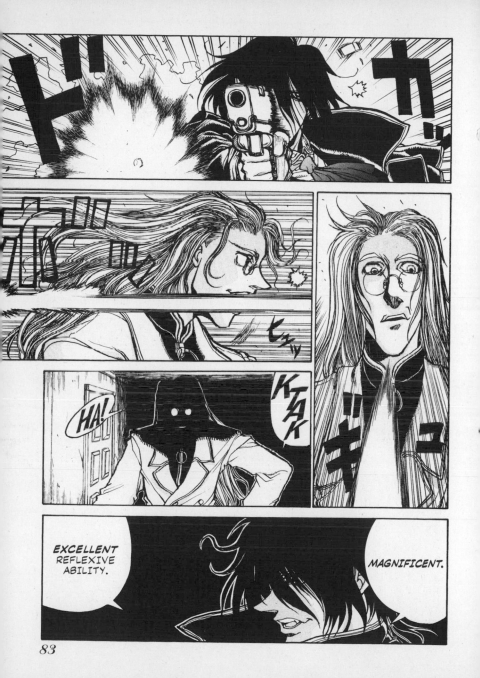

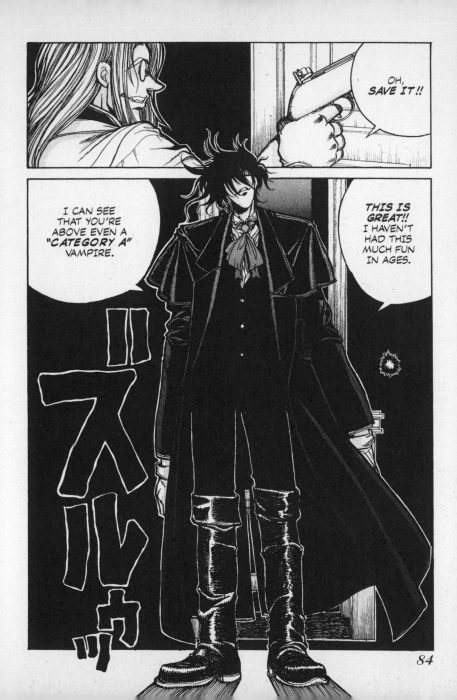

84

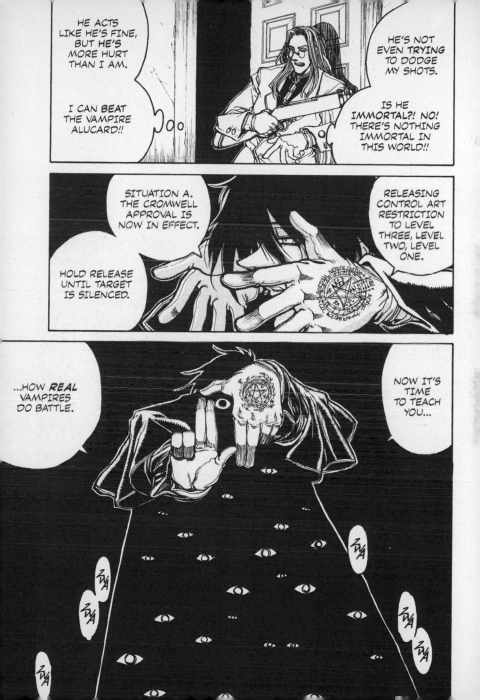

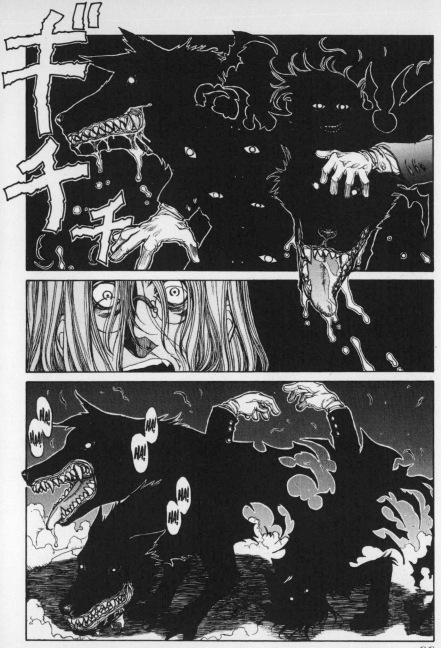

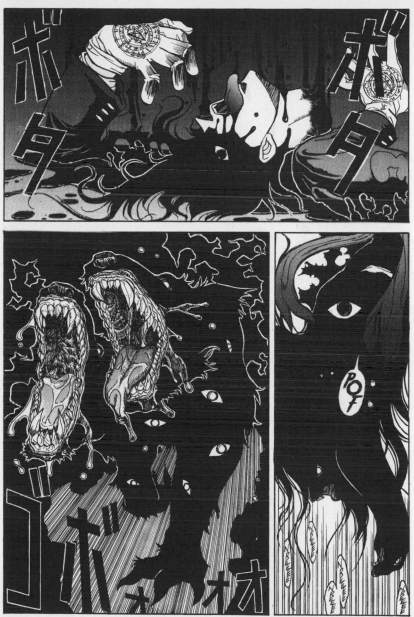

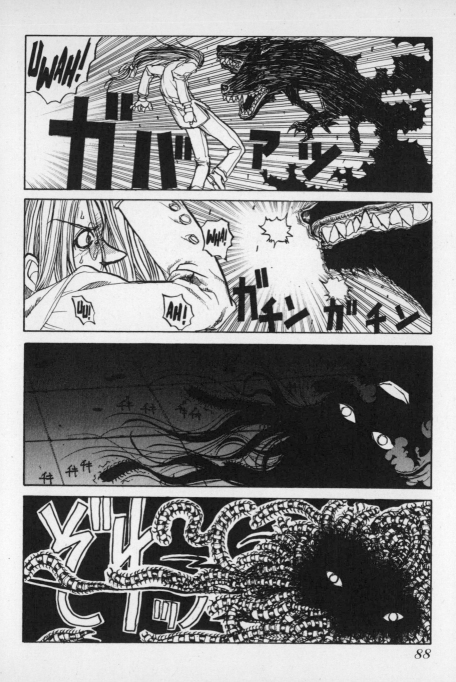

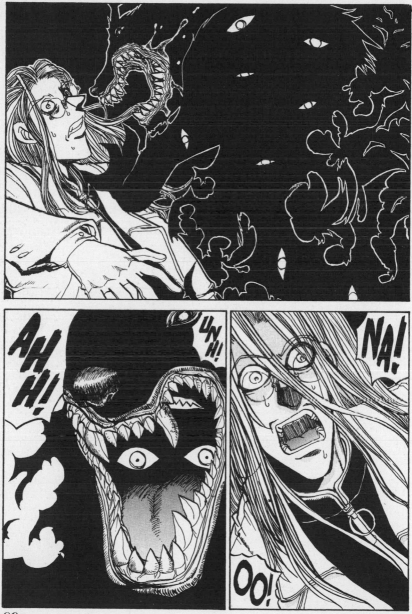

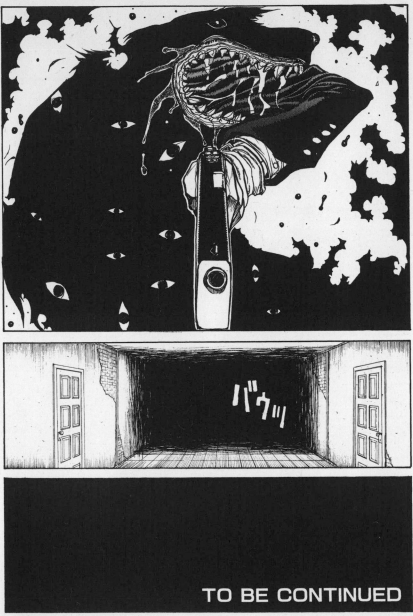

バウッ

TO BE CONTINUED

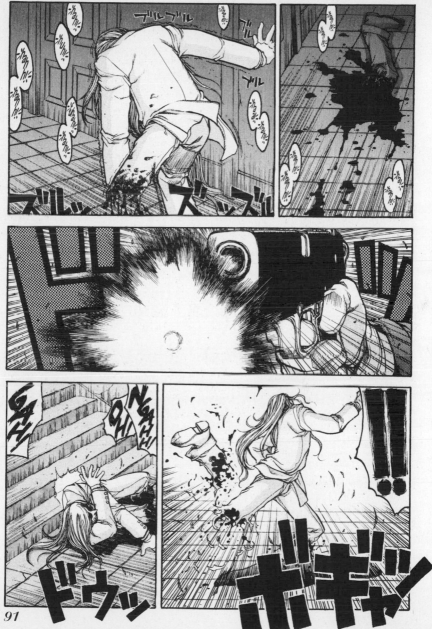

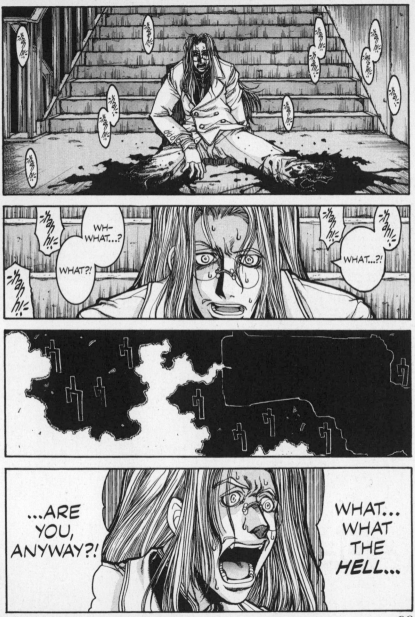

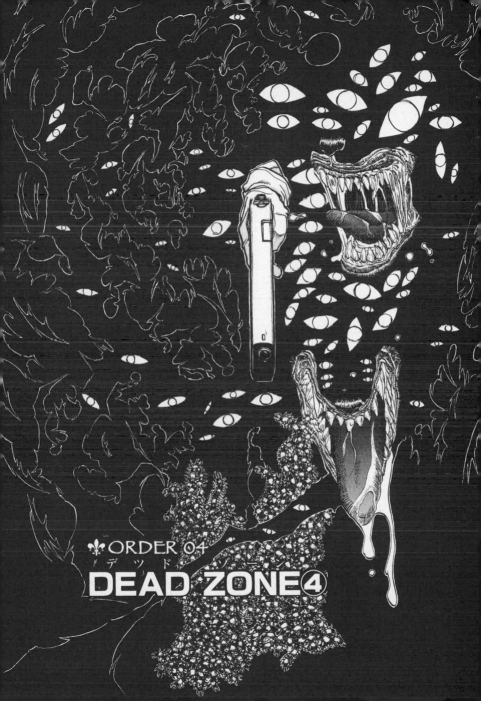

ORDER 04
DEAD ZONE④

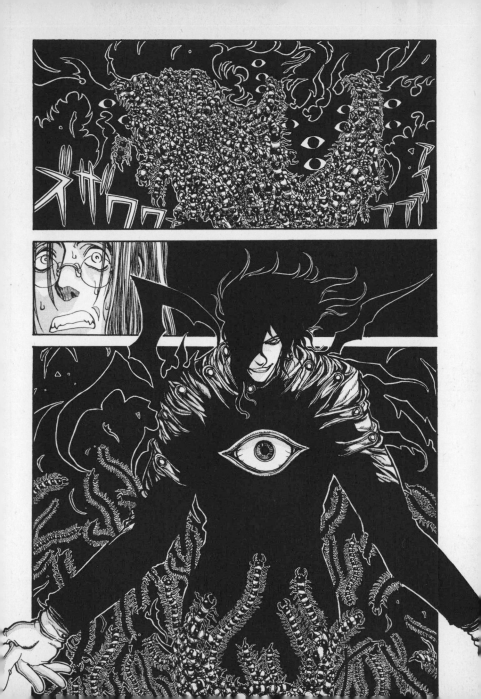

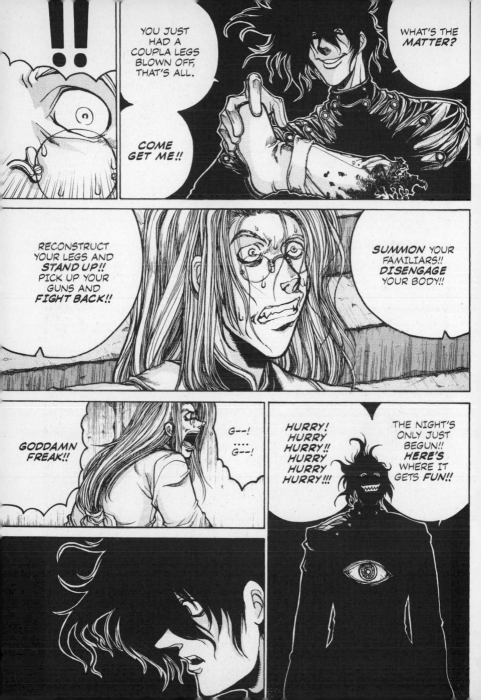

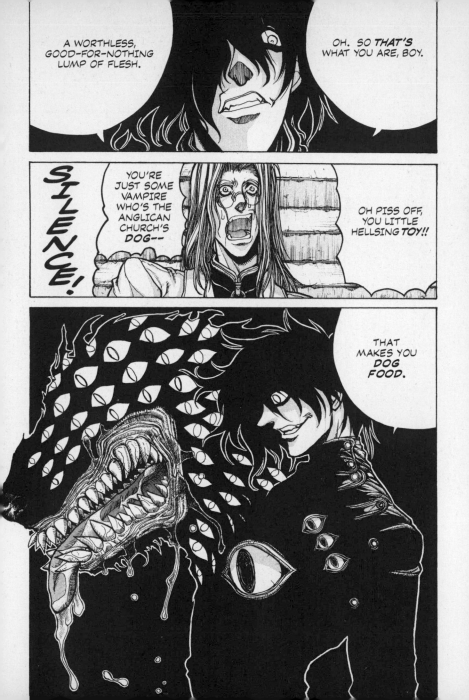

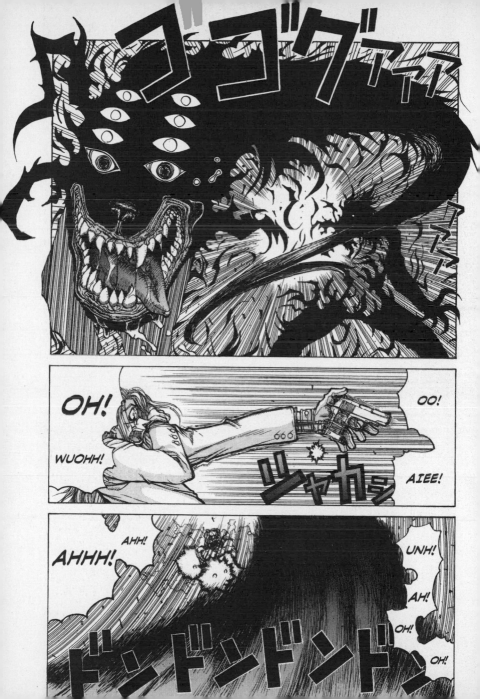

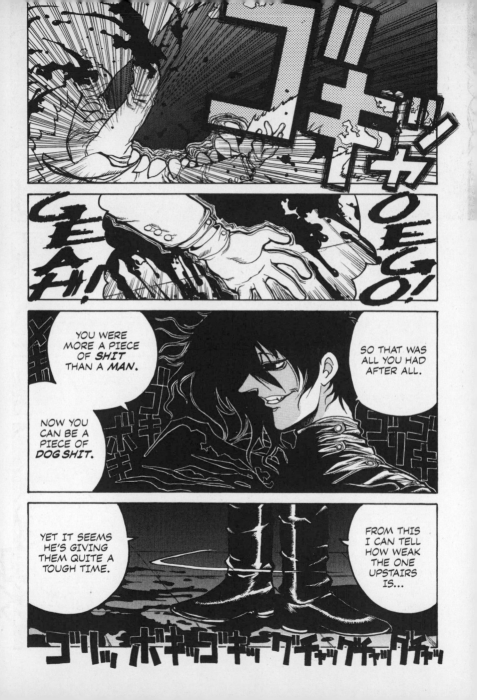

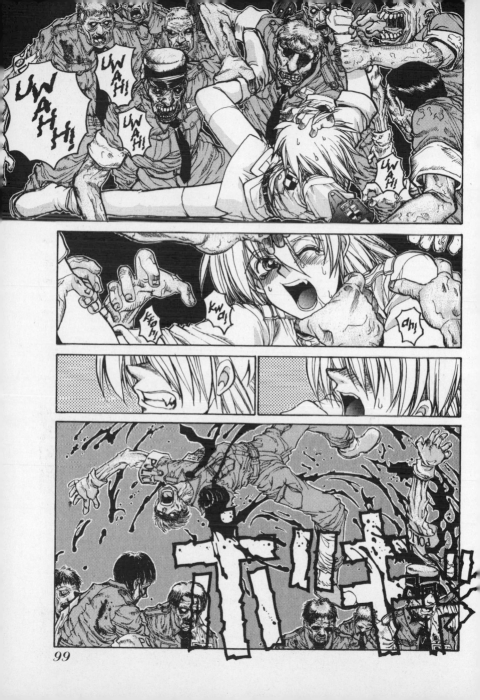

99

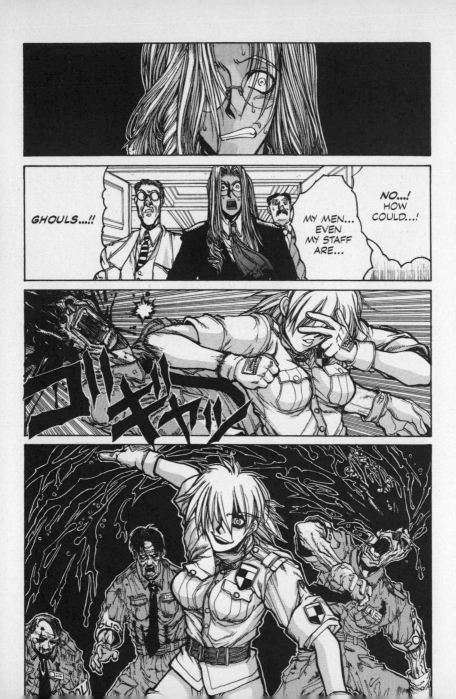

GHOULS....!!

MY MEN...
EVEN
MY STAFF
ARE...

NO....!
HOW
COULD...!

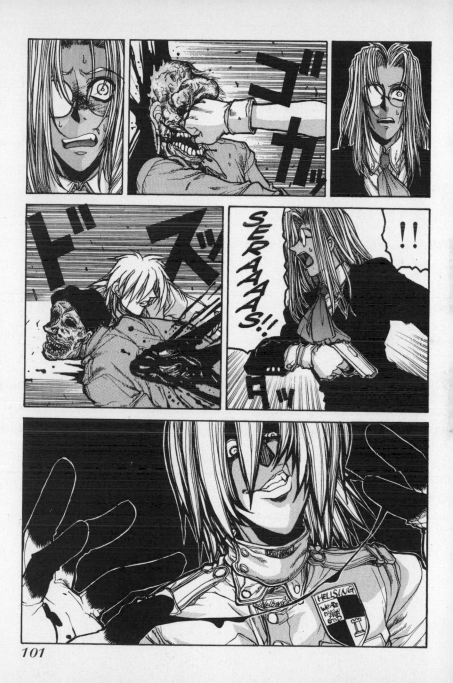

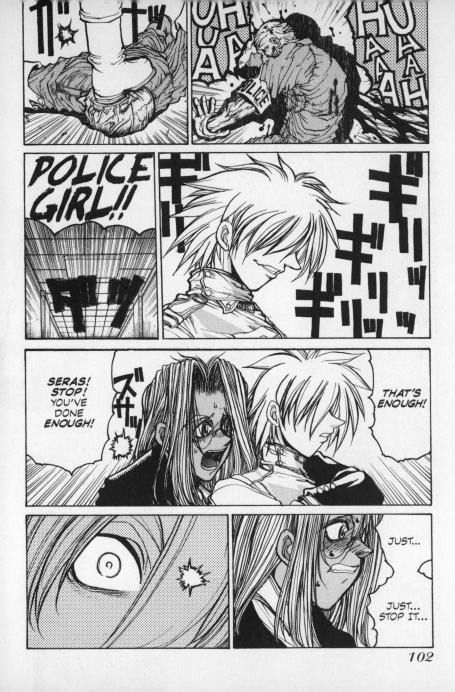

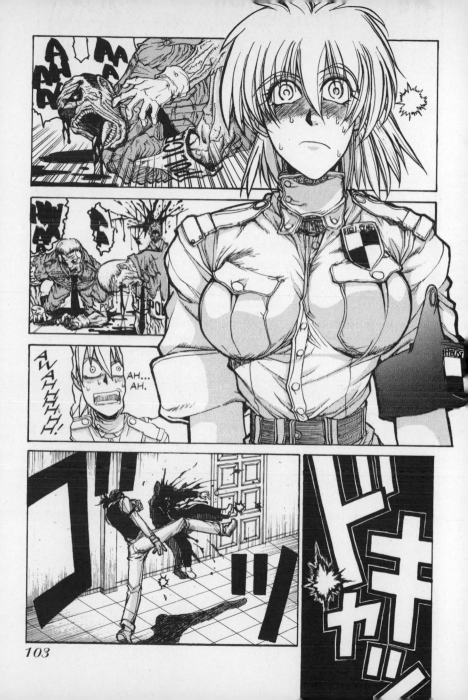

103

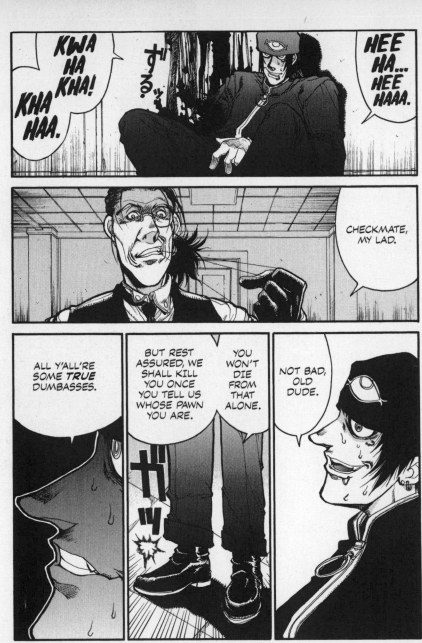

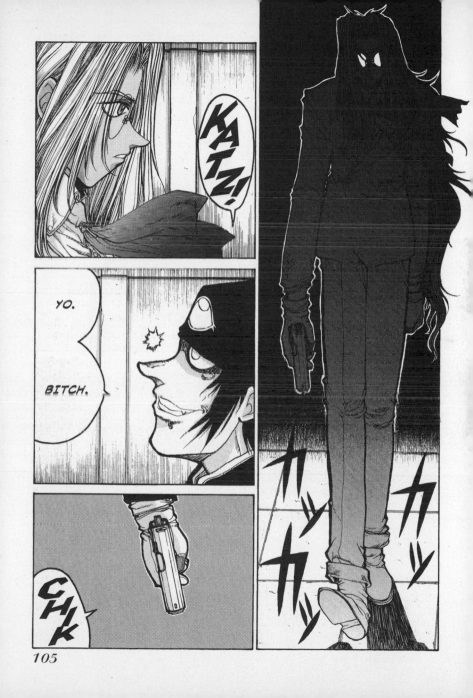

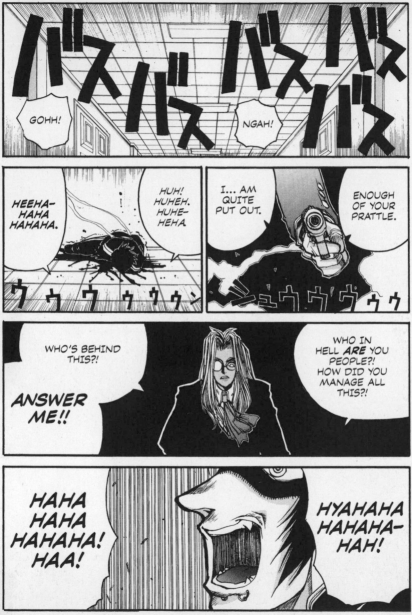

106

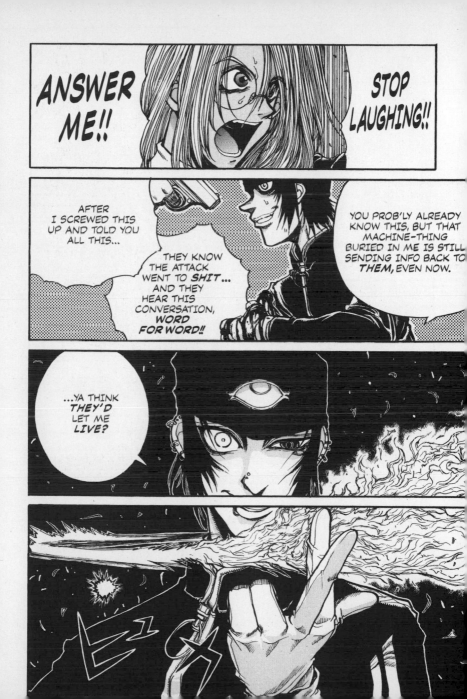

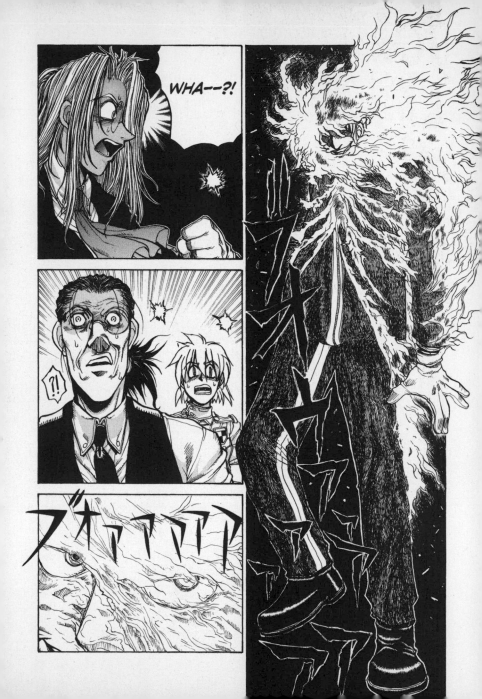

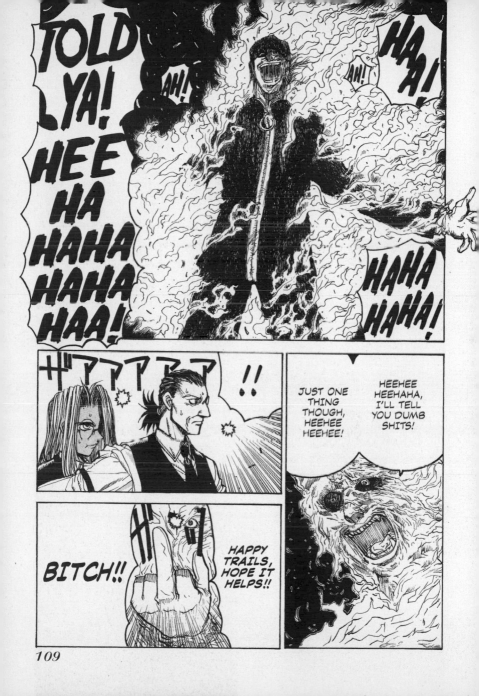

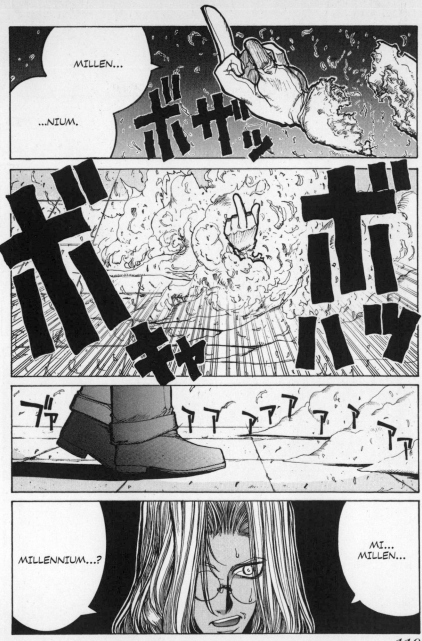

110

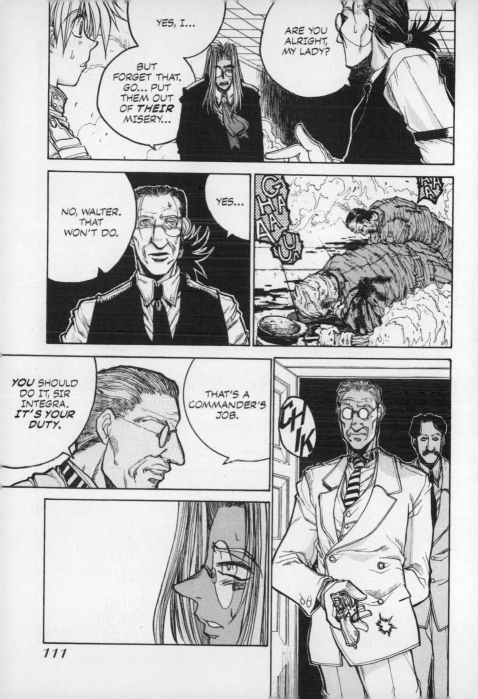

111

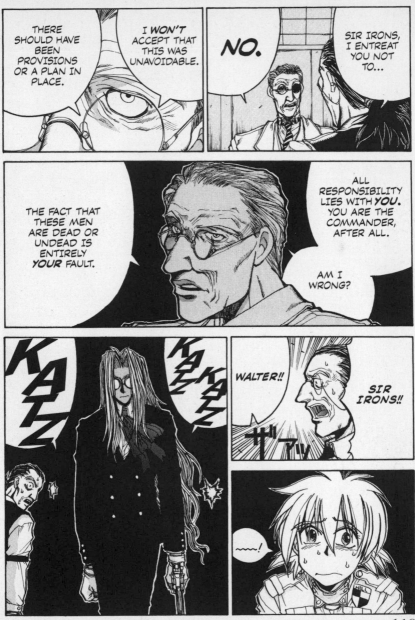

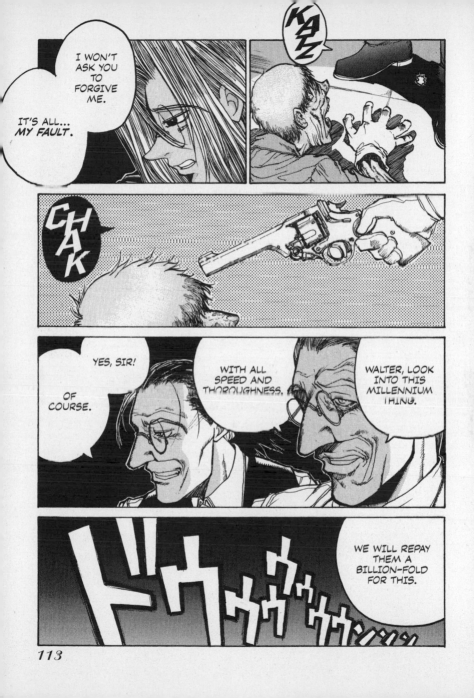

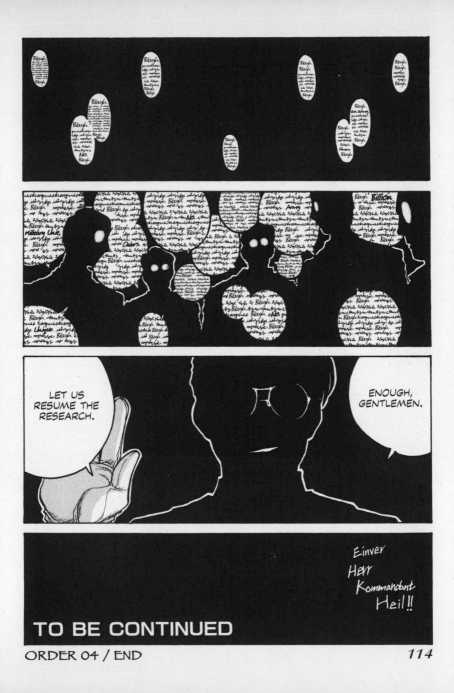

TO BE CONTINUED

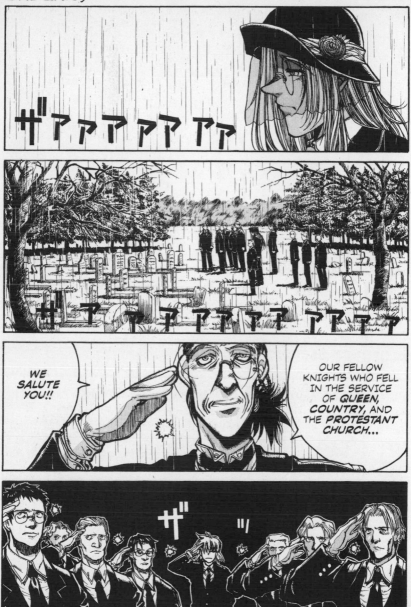

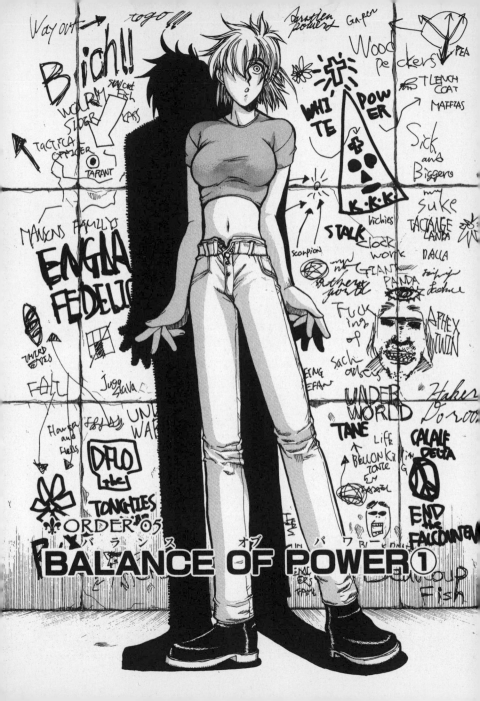

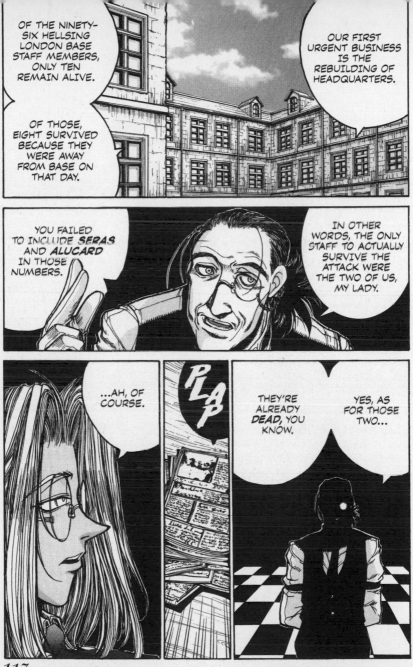

OF THE NINETY-SIX HELLSING LONDON BASE STAFF MEMBERS, ONLY TEN REMAIN ALIVE.

OUR FIRST URGENT BUSINESS IS THE REBUILDING OF HEADQUARTERS.

OF THOSE, EIGHT SURVIVED BECAUSE THEY WERE AWAY FROM BASE ON THAT DAY.

YOU FAILED TO INCLUDE *SERAS* AND *ALUCARD* IN THOSE NUMBERS.

IN OTHER WORDS, THE ONLY STAFF TO ACTUALLY SURVIVE THE ATTACK WERE THE TWO OF US, MY LADY.

...AH, OF COURSE.

PLAP

THEY'RE ALREADY *DEAD*, YOU KNOW.

YES, AS FOR THOSE TWO...

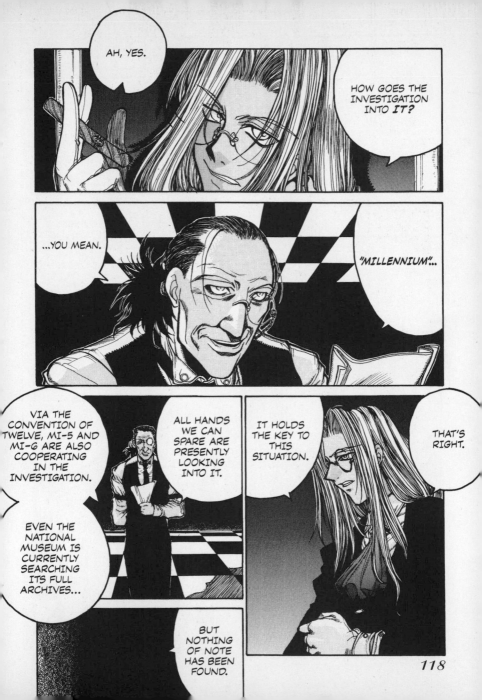

118

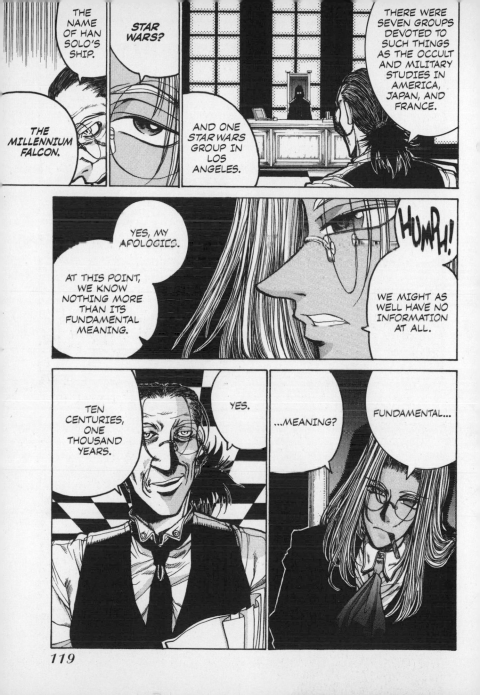

THE NAME OF HAN SOLO'S SHIP.

STAR WARS?

THERE WERE SEVEN GROUPS DEVOTED TO SUCH THINGS AS THE OCCULT AND MILITARY STUDIES IN AMERICA, JAPAN, AND FRANCE.

THE MILLENNIUM FALCON.

AND ONE STAR WARS GROUP IN LOS ANGELES.

YES, MY APOLOGIES.

AT THIS POINT, WE KNOW NOTHING MORE THAN ITS FUNDAMENTAL MEANING.

HUMPH!

WE MIGHT AS WELL HAVE NO INFORMATION AT ALL.

TEN CENTURIES, ONE THOUSAND YEARS.

YES.

...MEANING?

FUNDAMENTAL...

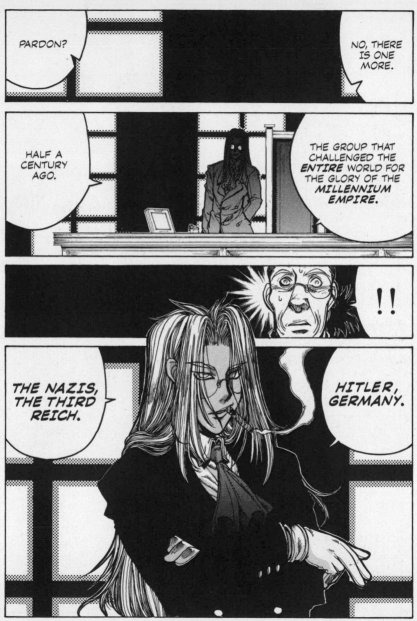

120

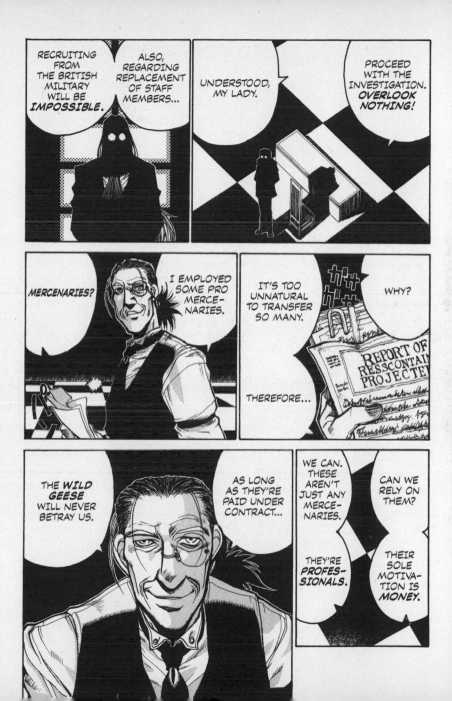

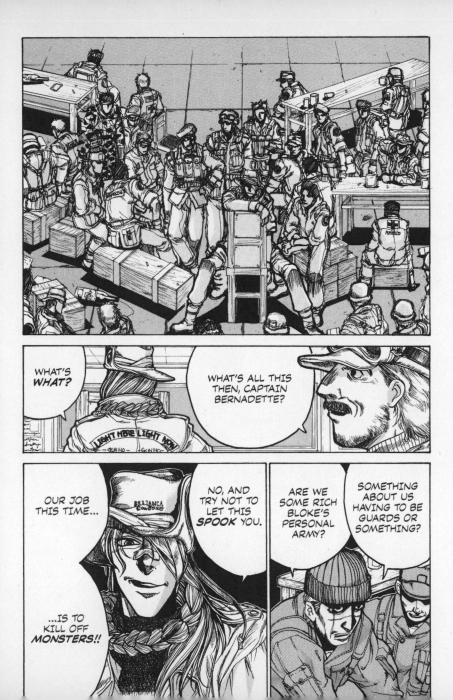

WHAT'S **WHAT?**

WHAT'S ALL THIS THEN, CAPTAIN BERNADETTE?

OUR JOB THIS TIME...

NO, AND TRY NOT TO LET THIS **SPOOK** YOU.

ARE WE SOME RICH BLOKE'S PERSONAL ARMY?

SOMETHING ABOUT US HAVING TO BE GUARDS OR SOMETHING?

...IS TO KILL OFF **MONSTERS!!**

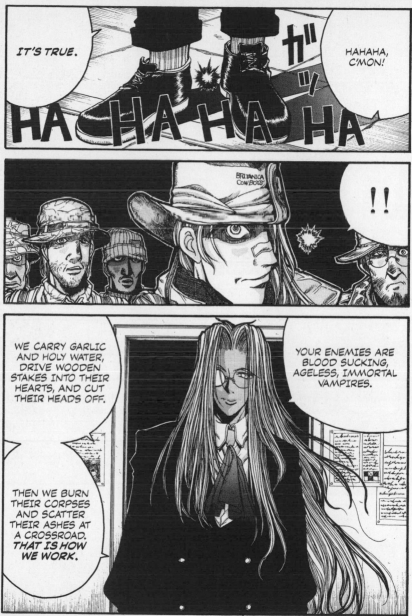

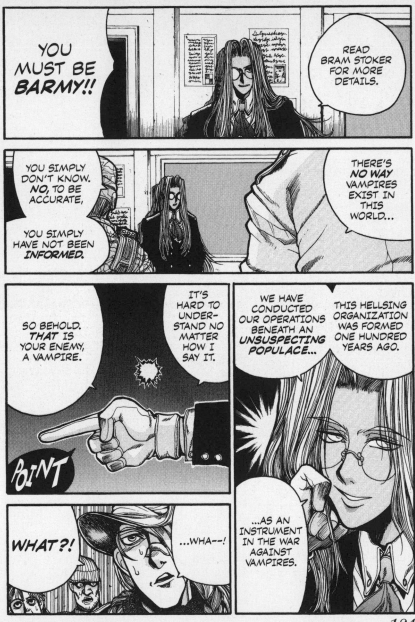

YOU MUST BE *BARMY!!*

READ BRAM STOKER FOR MORE DETAILS.

YOU SIMPLY DON'T KNOW. *NO,* TO BE ACCURATE,

YOU SIMPLY HAVE NOT BEEN *INFORMED.*

THERE'S *NO WAY* VAMPIRES EXIST IN THIS WORLD...

SO BEHOLD. *THAT* IS YOUR ENEMY, A VAMPIRE.

IT'S HARD TO UNDERSTAND NO MATTER HOW I SAY IT.

WE HAVE CONDUCTED OUR OPERATIONS BENEATH AN *UNSUSPECTING POPULACE...*

THIS HELLSING ORGANIZATION WAS FORMED ONE HUNDRED YEARS AGO.

POINT

...AS AN INSTRUMENT IN THE WAR AGAINST VAMPIRES.

WHAT?!

...WHA--!

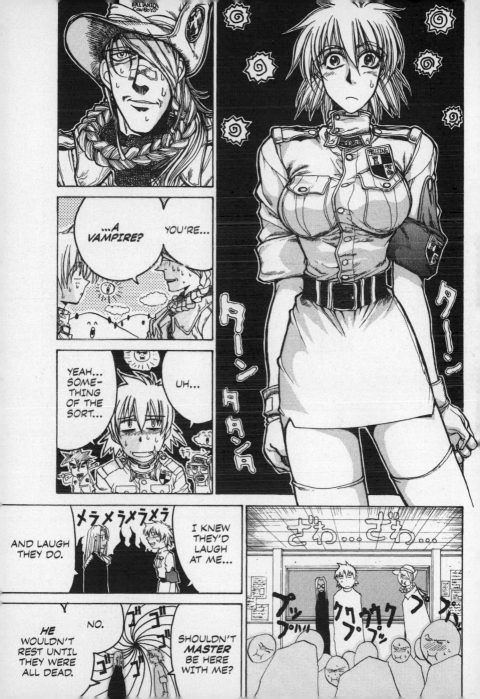

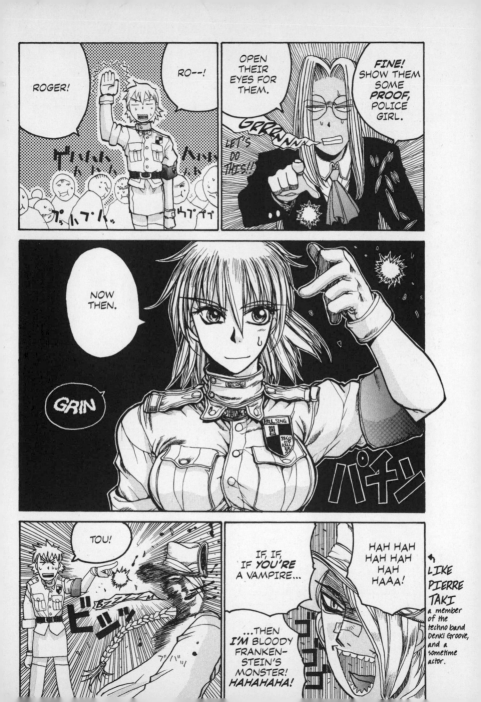

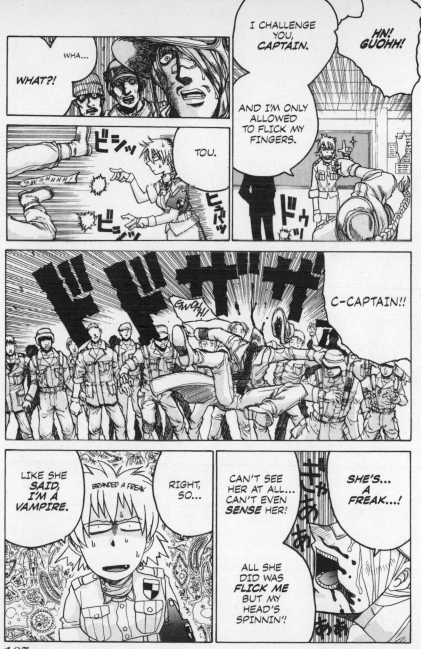

127

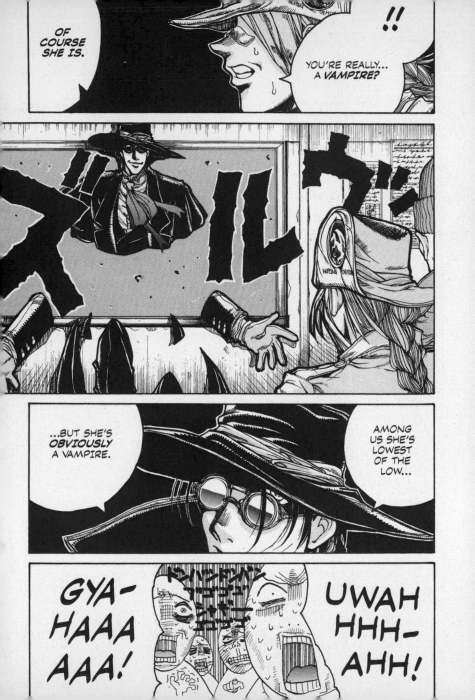

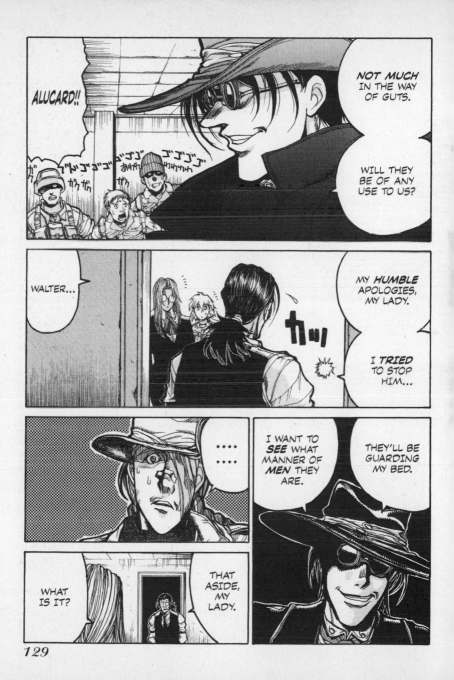

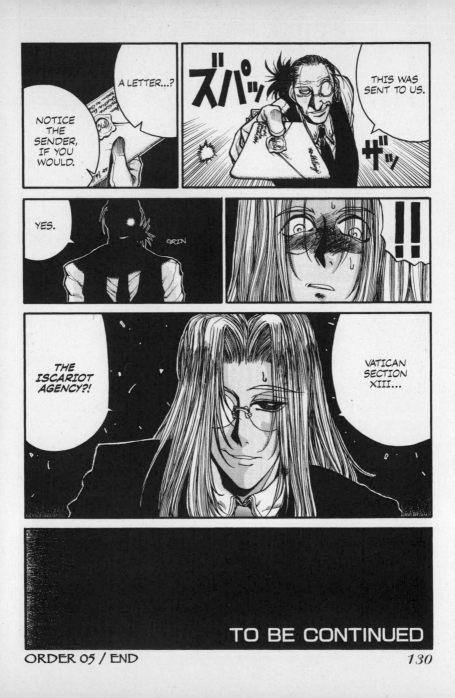

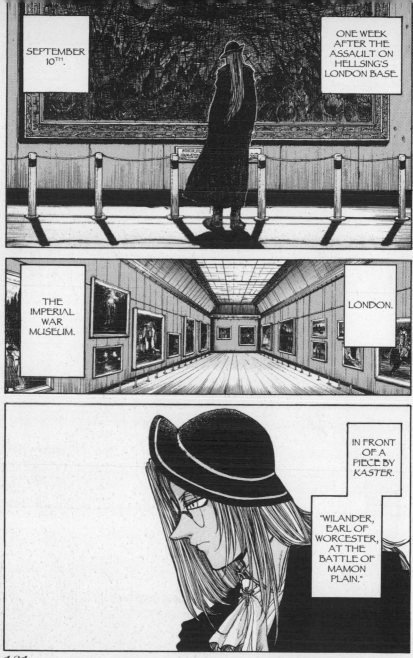

SEPTEMBER 10TH.

ONE WEEK AFTER THE ASSAULT ON HELLSING'S LONDON BASE.

THE IMPERIAL WAR MUSEUM.

LONDON.

IN FRONT OF A PIECE BY KASTER.

"WILANDER, EARL OF WORCESTER, AT THE BATTLE OF MAMON PLAIN."

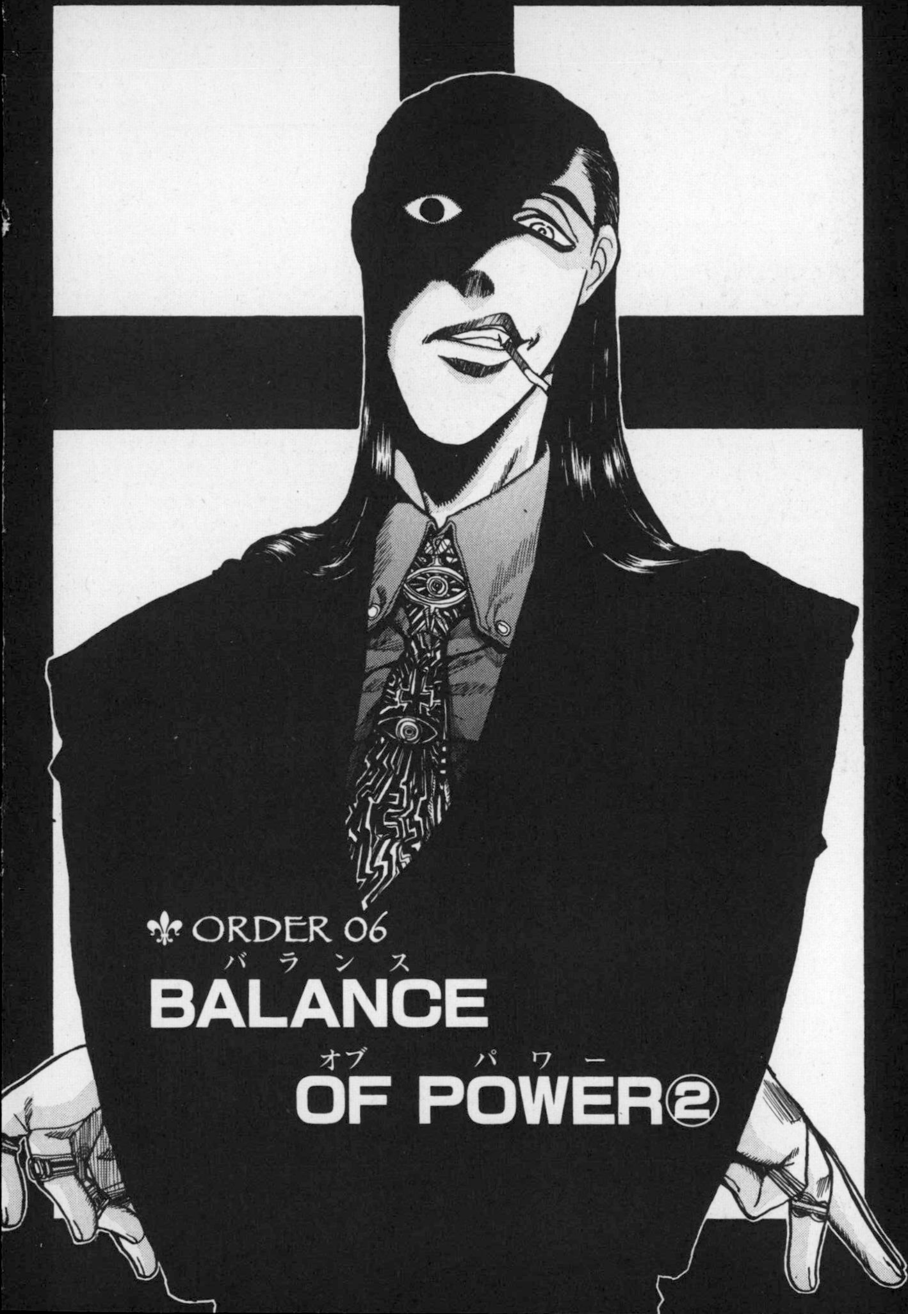

ORDER 06
バランス
BALANCE
オブ　パワー
OF POWER②

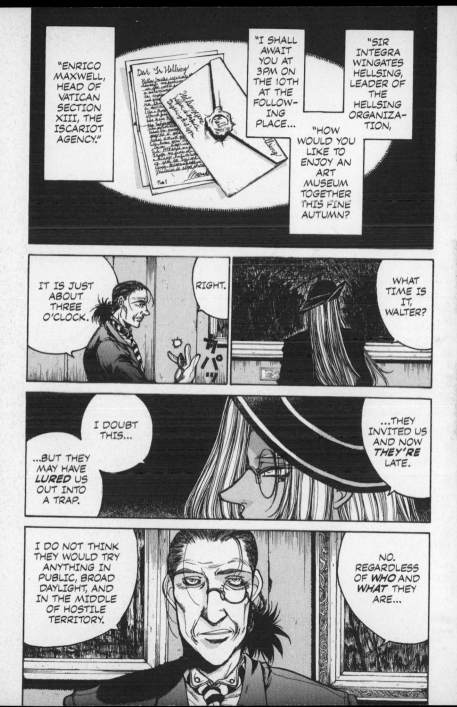

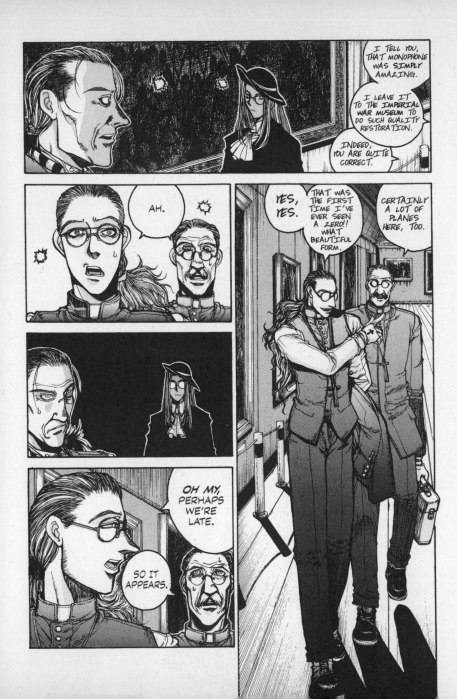

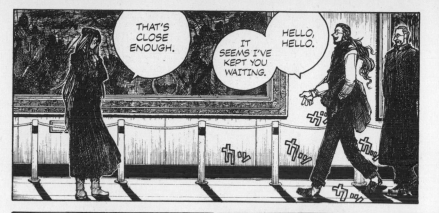

THAT'S CLOSE ENOUGH.

IT SEEMS I'VE KEPT YOU WAITING.

HELLO, HELLO.

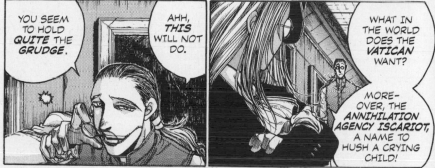

YOU SEEM TO HOLD *QUITE* THE *GRUDGE*.

AHH, *THIS* WILL NOT DO.

WHAT IN THE WORLD DOES THE *VATICAN* WANT?

MORE-OVER, THE *ANNIHILATION AGENCY ISCARIOT*, A NAME TO HUSH A CRYING CHILD!

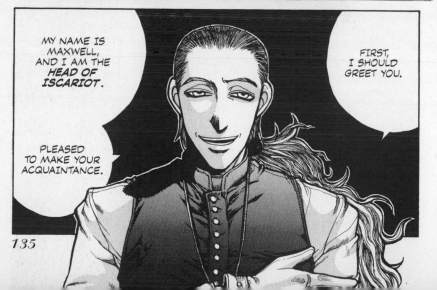

MY NAME IS MAXWELL, AND I AM THE *HEAD OF ISCARIOT*.

FIRST, I SHOULD GREET YOU.

PLEASED TO MAKE YOUR ACQUAINTANCE.

135

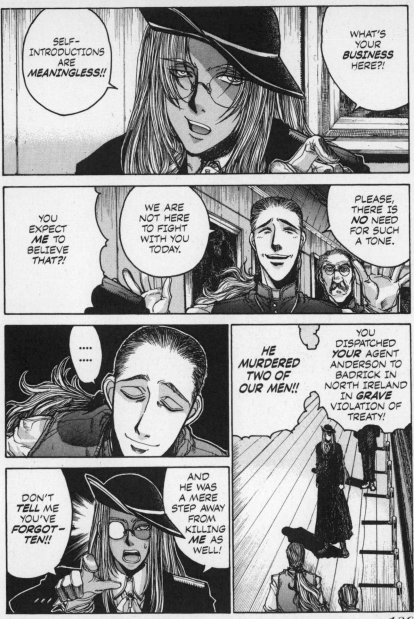

136

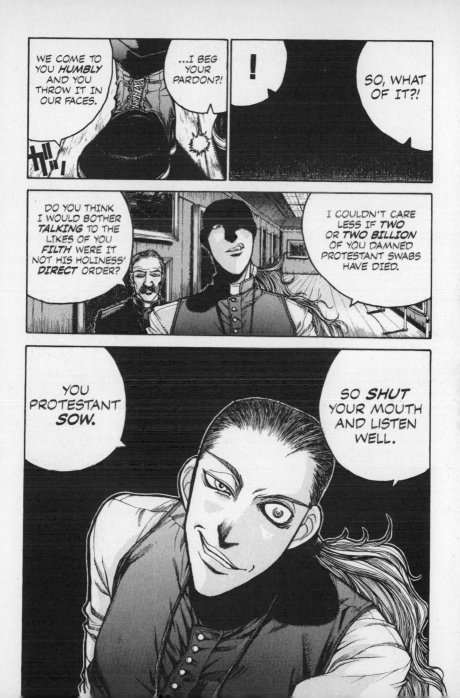

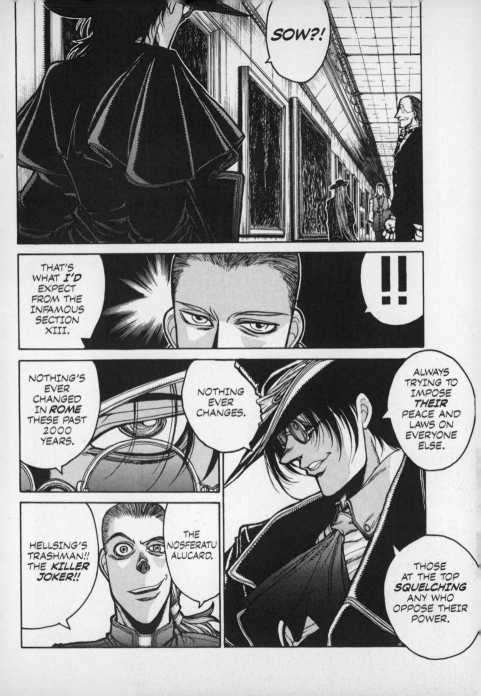

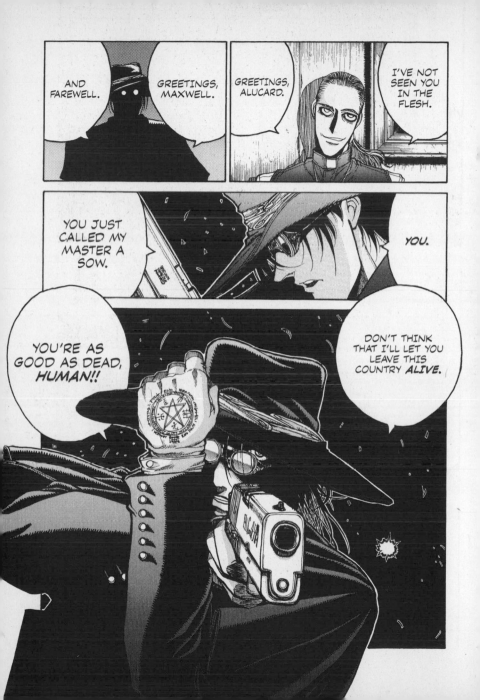

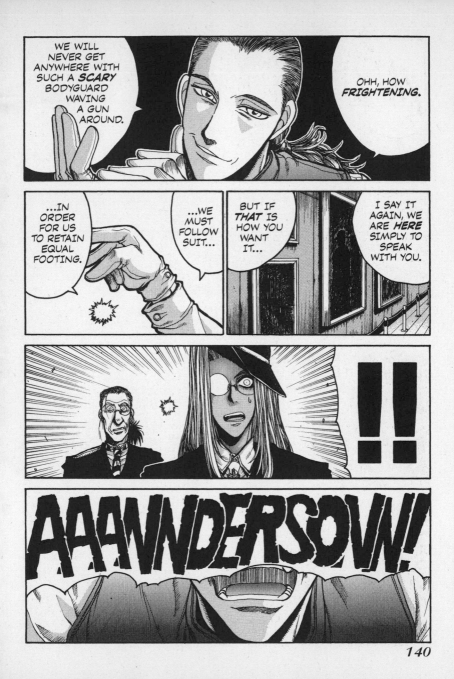

140

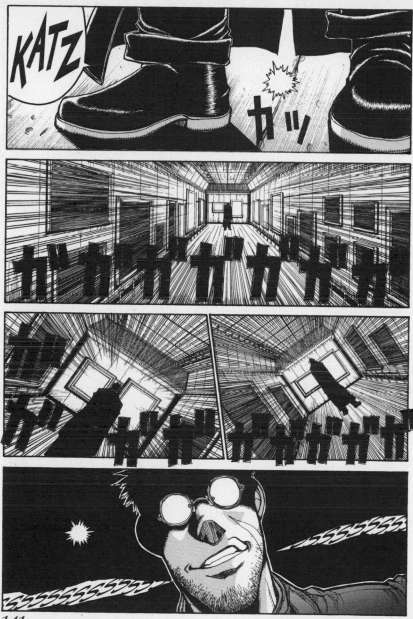

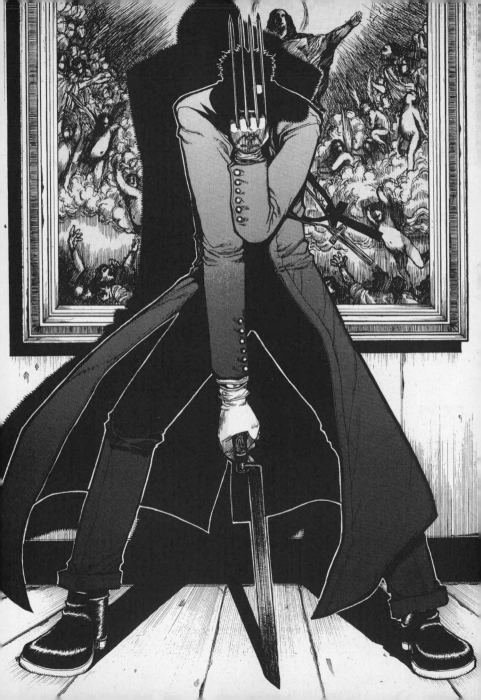

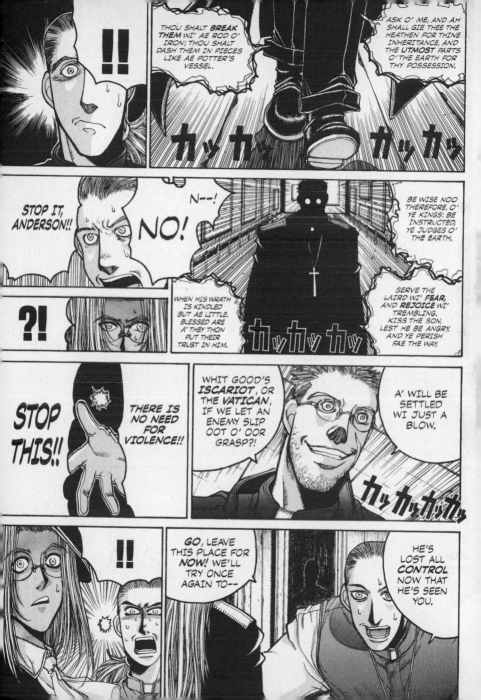

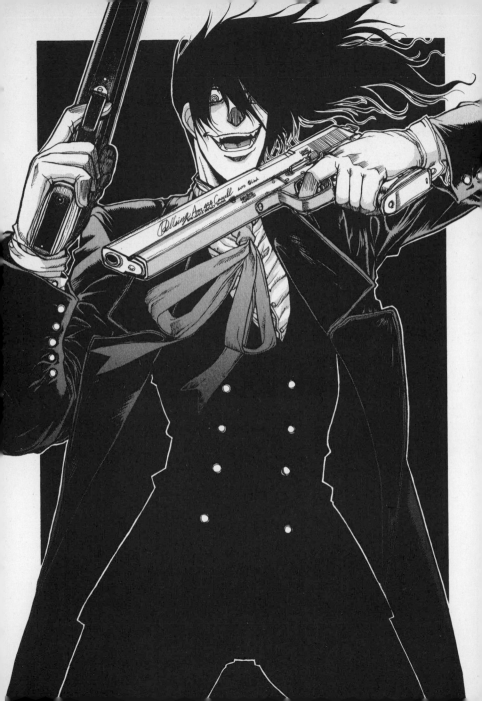

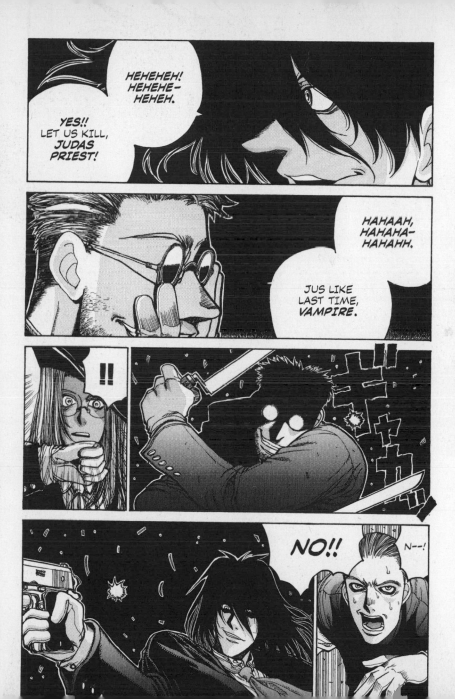

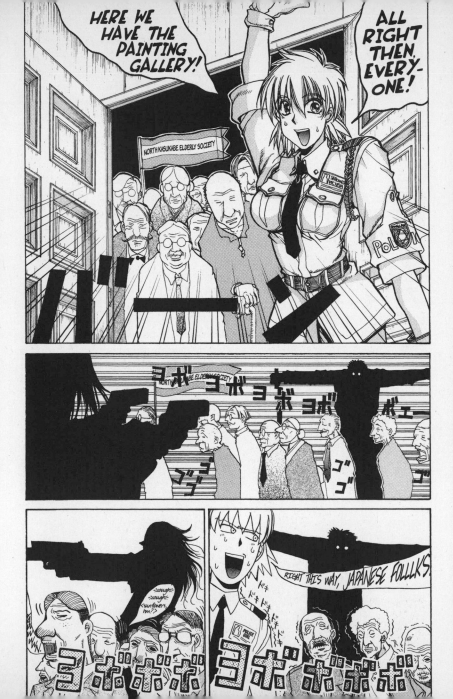

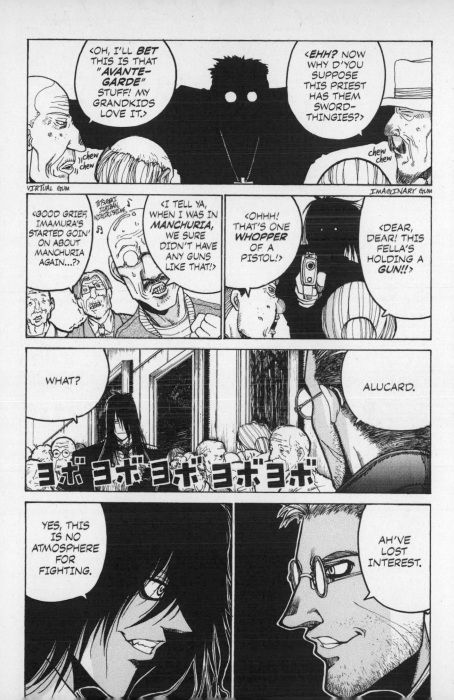

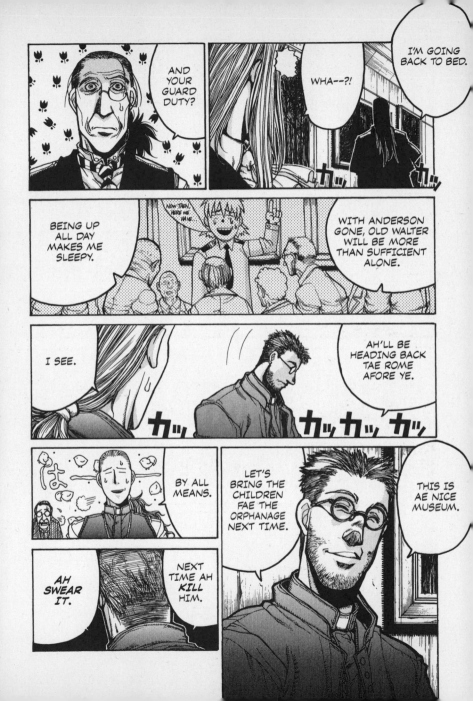

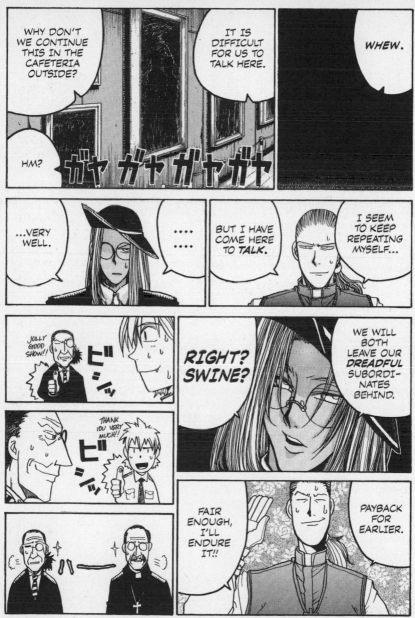

149

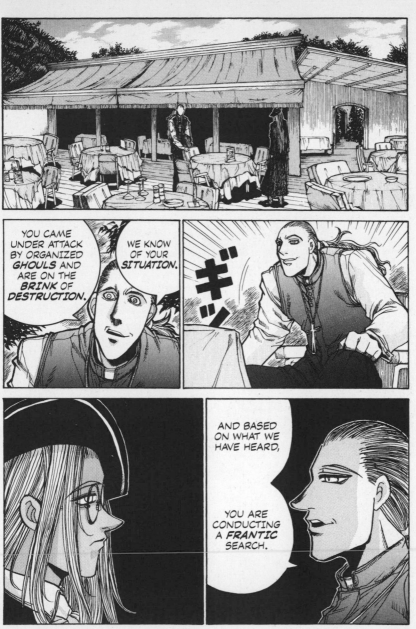

YOU CAME UNDER ATTACK BY ORGANIZED *GHOULS* AND ARE ON THE *BRINK* OF *DESTRUCTION.*

WE KNOW OF YOUR *SITUATION.*

ギッ

AND BASED ON WHAT WE HAVE HEARD,

YOU ARE CONDUCTING A *FRANTIC* SEARCH.

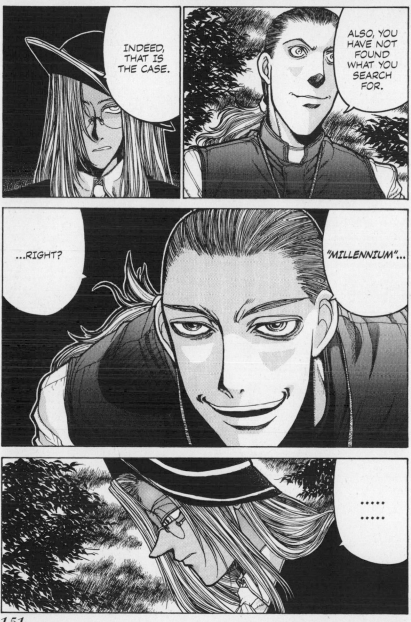

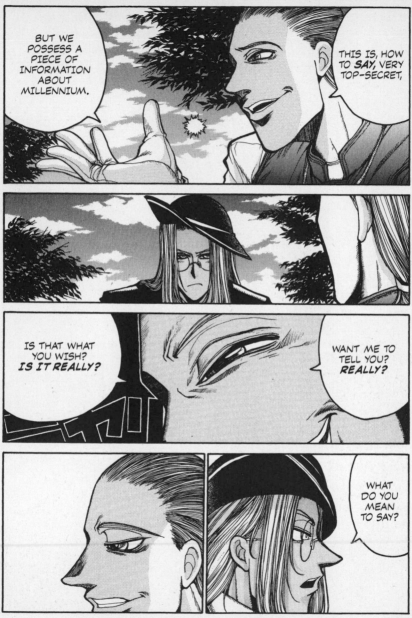

152

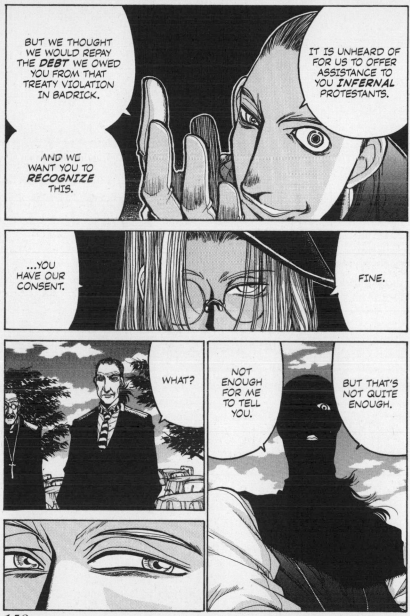

BUT WE THOUGHT WE WOULD REPAY THE *DEBT* WE OWED YOU FROM THAT TREATY VIOLATION IN BADRICK.

IT IS UNHEARD OF FOR US TO OFFER ASSISTANCE TO YOU *INFERNAL* PROTESTANTS.

AND WE WANT YOU TO *RECOGNIZE* THIS.

...YOU HAVE OUR CONSENT.

FINE.

WHAT?

NOT ENOUGH FOR ME TO TELL YOU.

BUT THAT'S NOT QUITE ENOUGH.

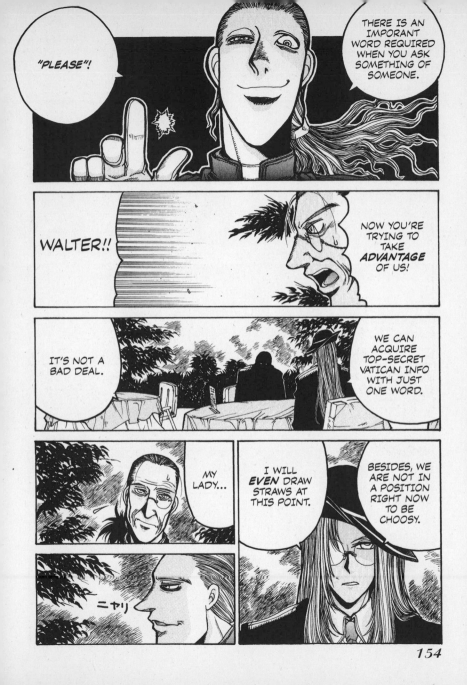

154

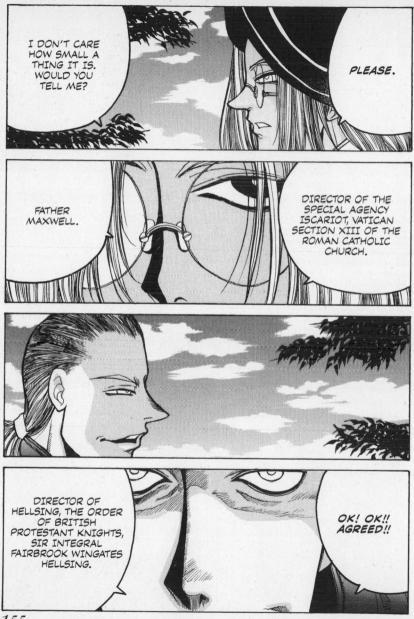

155

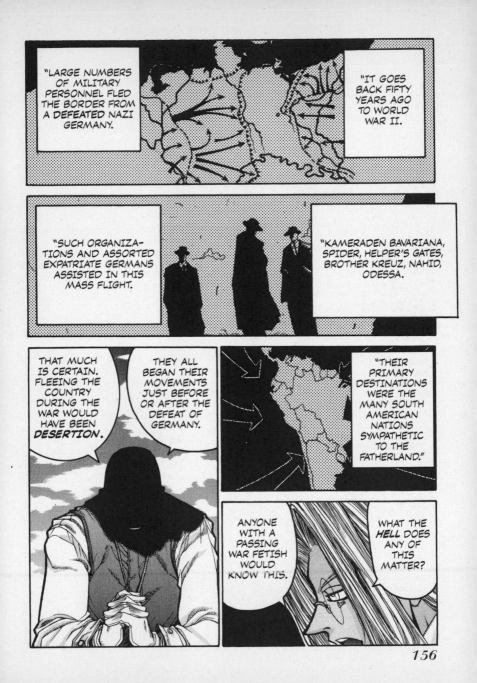

"LARGE NUMBERS OF MILITARY PERSONNEL FLED THE BORDER FROM A DEFEATED NAZI GERMANY.

"IT GOES BACK FIFTY YEARS AGO TO WORLD WAR II.

"SUCH ORGANIZA-TIONS AND ASSORTED EXPATRIATE GERMANS ASSISTED IN THIS MASS FLIGHT.

"KAMERADEN BAVARIANA, SPIDER, HELPER'S GATES, BROTHER KREUZ, NAHID, ODESSA.

THAT MUCH IS CERTAIN. FLEEING THE COUNTRY DURING THE WAR WOULD HAVE BEEN *DESERTION*.

THEY ALL BEGAN THEIR MOVEMENTS JUST BEFORE OR AFTER THE DEFEAT OF GERMANY.

"THEIR PRIMARY DESTINATIONS WERE THE MANY SOUTH AMERICAN NATIONS SYMPATHETIC TO THE FATHERLAND."

ANYONE WITH A PASSING WAR FETISH WOULD KNOW THIS.

WHAT THE *HELL* DOES ANY OF THIS MATTER?

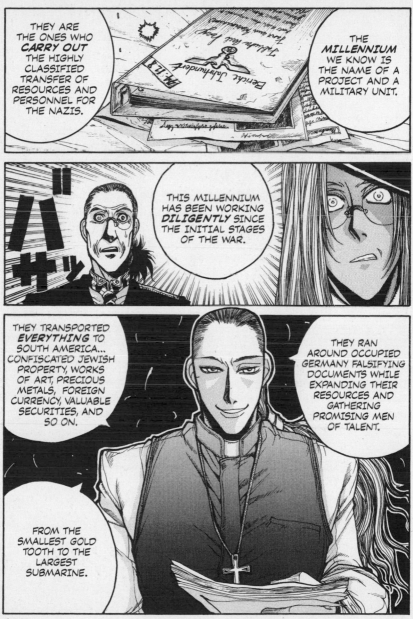

THEY ARE THE ONES WHO **CARRY OUT** THE HIGHLY CLASSIFIED TRANSFER OF RESOURCES AND PERSONNEL FOR THE NAZIS.

THE **MILLENNIUM** WE KNOW IS THE NAME OF A PROJECT AND A MILITARY UNIT.

THIS MILLENNIUM HAS BEEN WORKING **DILIGENTLY** SINCE THE INITIAL STAGES OF THE WAR.

THEY TRANSPORTED **EVERYTHING** TO SOUTH AMERICA... CONFISCATED JEWISH PROPERTY, WORKS OF ART, PRECIOUS METALS, FOREIGN CURRENCY, VALUABLE SECURITIES, AND SO ON.

THEY RAN AROUND OCCUPIED GERMANY FALSIFYING DOCUMENTS WHILE EXPANDING THEIR RESOURCES AND GATHERING PROMISING MEN OF TALENT.

FROM THE SMALLEST GOLD TOOTH TO THE LARGEST SUBMARINE.

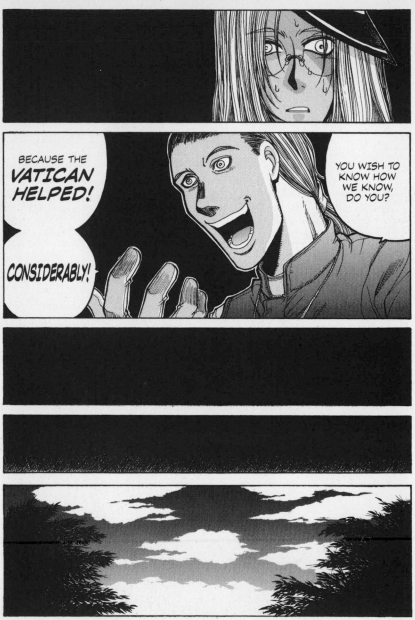

158

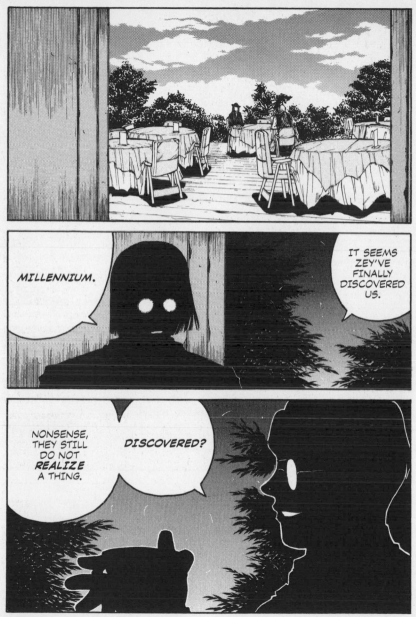

159

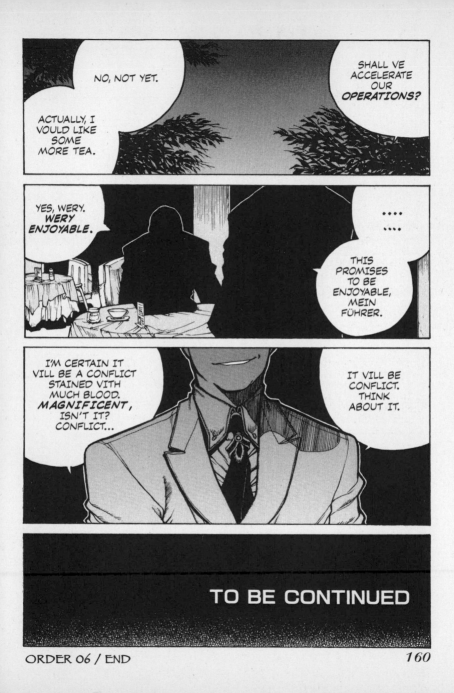

hiranokohta

■ YEAHHH. CHINKO CHINKO! (MY GREETING) GOOD EVENING. THIS IS KOHTA HIRANO. AND SO HERE IT IS FINALLY, HELLSING VOLUME 2. IT'S LIKE, "PUB-LIIIIIISH!!" OR SOMETHING. IT ENDED UP TAKING MORE THAN A WHOLE YEAR TO GET IT RELEASED. AND IT'S LEFT ME EXHAUSTED. IT WAS ROUGH! I'M ALL WORN OUT. I'M KAORU KUROKI. IT'S A SEXUAL RELEASE. TOOOOT TOOOOOT (PROUDLY SHOWING OFF HER ARMPITS WHILE PLAYING A LITTLE CONCH SHELL) TOOOOT TOOOOT TOOOOT TOOOOT TOOOO1 TOOO1

*note: Kaoru Kuroki was an actress in the 80's, famous for not shaving her armpits. She was also known to talk about the idea of sexual release a lot.

■ AND SO, CHARACTERS FROM MY ADULT BOOKS WILL SHOW UP. NAZIS WILL SHOW UP. SINCE VOLUME 1 I'VE BEEN ABLE TO DO ABSOLUTELY WHATEVER I PLEASE, BUT YOU KNOW, IT'S KIND OF LIKE SOME RAMEN SHOP OWNED AND RUN BY ONE GUY AND THE RAMEN IS TERRRRIBLE. NO MATTER WHAT ANYONE SAYS HE DOESN'T GIVE THEM THE TIME OF DAY AND KEEPS SERVING CRAPULENT RAMEN. SO ALL I CAN SAY IS I'M SORRY IT ALL SEEMS SO WEIRD AND DARK.

■ THERE WAS A LOT OF FOCUS ON OLD MEN IN THIS VOLUME AND IT PROBABLY SEEMS FISHY AND UNBALANCED TO THE READERS. ALL I CAN SAY IS I'M SORRY.

■ IN ANY CASE, FROM HERE ON THE STORY WILL GO ON "DAAAARA DAAAARA," AND IT'D MAKE ME HAPPY IF ALL OF YOU READ IT "DAAAARA DAAAARA." BUT THEN I GUESS IT'S ALREADY THAT WAY ANYWAY. DARAAAA DARAAAA. MIDARA-AAA MIDARAAAA! NOOO NOOO NOOO NOOO! IT'S TEN DARAAAA. (SOUNDING LIKE TAKAYANAGI FROM SMAP)

*note: you're going to have to figure this stuff out on your own!

■ ZZ GUNDAM IS PRETTY COOL...
I WONDER IF ROUX LOUKA WOULD BE
WILLING TO MARRY ME...

■ MAYBE I WISH MRS. DEVI WOULD JUST DIE.
MARIANNE, TOO.

*note: Two Japanese celebrities who have been known to hold grudges against each other. Think afternoon talk-show fare.

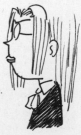

~ THE IDIOT BROTHERS ~

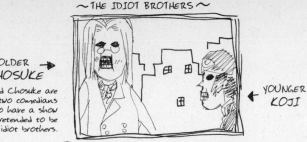

OLDER **CHOSUKE** →

*note: Koji and Chosuke are the names of two comedians who used to have a show where they pretended to be idiot brothers.

← YOUNGER **KOJI**

⊙ (USELESS) CHARACTER DESCRIPTIONS

■ JAN VALENTINE

HE GOT BURNED TO A CRISP. BWOOOSH. I **DREW** ALL THOSE PIERCINGS AND EVEN I THOUGHT THEY LOOKED PAINFUL. I KEPT THINKING "WHO ARE YOU, KAKI-HARA?!" OF COURSE, IF THEY MISS IT'LL BE A COCK PIERCING. TWO OF THEM, EVEN. "AT THIS POINT, THE DOG'S THE ONLY ONE NOT FREAKIN' OUT." GINYAAA! GOOD-BYE, JAN VALENTINE.

*note: Kakihara is a character from the movie "Ichi the Killer," and has lots of facial metal.

■ LUKE VALENTINE

GUESS HE WAS TOO MUCH FORM OVER FUNCTION. HE DOESN'T DESERVE TO WEAR ROUND GLASSES. AND YOU KNOW, THAT'S IT! IN TERMS OF SAINT SEIYA, HE'S KIND OF LIKE CANCER DEATHMASK I GUESS. "SEKISHIKI MEIKAI HAAAA!" "I'M DROPPING YOU STRAIGHT DOWN THE YOMOTSU HIRASAKA!" GYAPIII! GOOD-BYE, LUKE VALENTINE.

*note: The Japanese attack shouted out above translates to "Cancer Hades Wave." The Yomotsu Hirasaka is a cliff or slope said to be on the pathway to Hades in Japanese mythology. This is an actual scene in the Saint Seiya series.

■ DIRECTOR MAXWELL

HE ALSO APPEARED IN CROSS FIRE, BUT HE LOOKED TOO MUCH LIKE INTEGRA SO I SLICKED HIS HAIR BACK. ALSO HAD HIM LOSE HIS GLASSES. THEN, SAY WHAT?! HE'S LIKE A WHOLE OTHER CHARACTER. IF I DON'T DO ANYTHING TO DIF-FERENTIATE MY CHARACTERS, IT LEADS TO REALIZATION. LETDOWN. DISAPPOINTMENT. INCONTINENCE. BLOODY STOOL. FAINTING. DEATH. HEAVEN. REINCARNATION. HI, I'M BACK.

■ DARK SHADOWS MAN

HE'S A VILLIAN SO HE GETS LOTS OF DARK SHADING.

◀ CROSS FIRE PART 2...COMMONLY KNOWN AS ROSS; FA FOR SHORT.

NOT ENOUGH! THERE AREN'T ENOUGH PAGES!! AND SO, CONTINUING ON FROM VOLUME I, THIS IS PART 2 OF THE STORY. HERE FOLLOWS THE SECOND ONE-SHOT INSTALLMENT IN WHICH MEMBERS OF THE VATICAN SPECIALIZED SECRET AGENCY SECTION XIII ISCARIOT ARE THE MAIN CHARACTERS. THE ART AND STORY ARE BOTH KIND OF ROUGH AND CRUDE SO I ASK THAT YOU BE UNDERSTANDING ABOUT THAT.

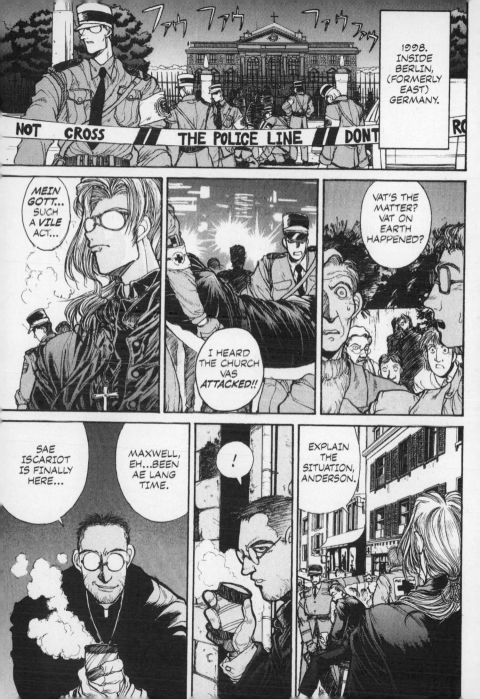

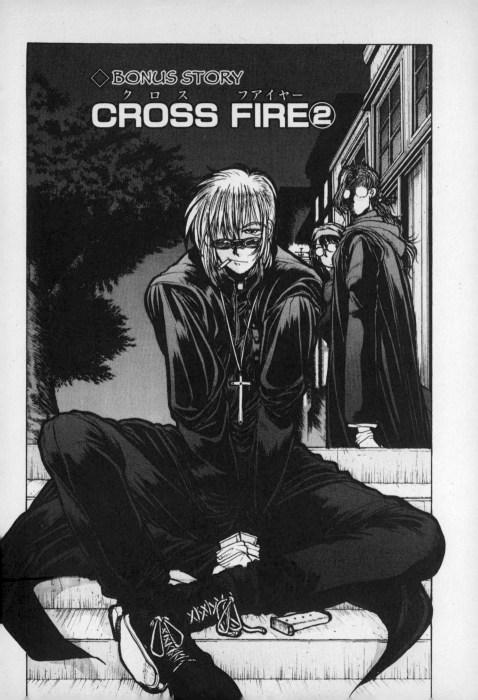

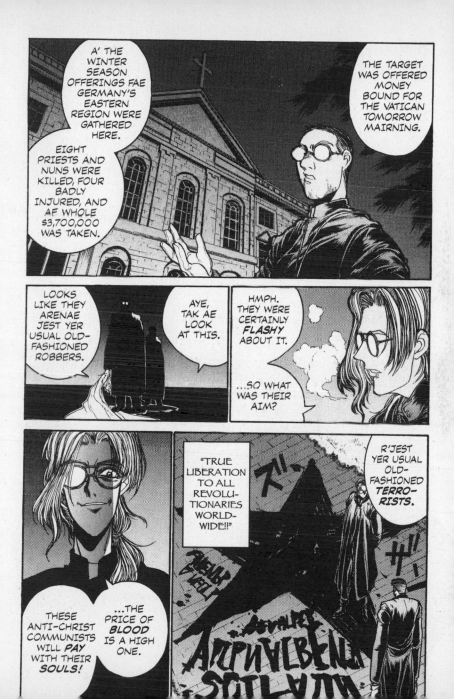

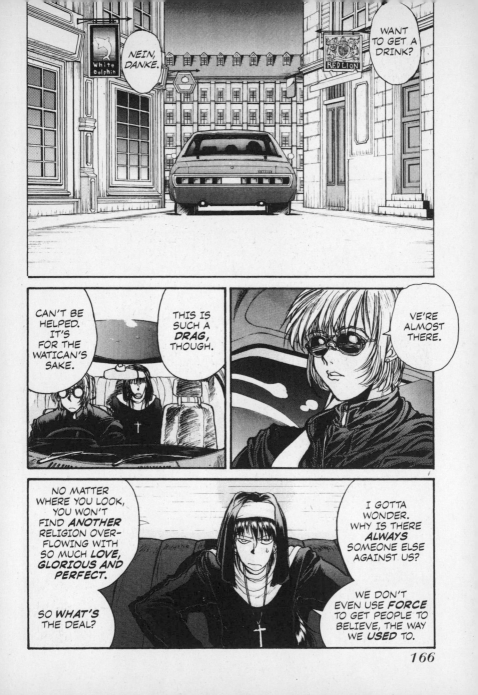

166

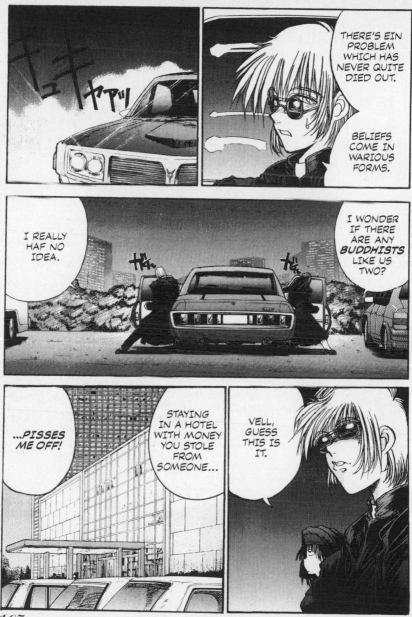

THERE'S EIN PROBLEM WHICH HAS NEVER QUITE DIED OUT.

BELIEFS COME IN WARIOUS FORMS.

I WONDER IF THERE ARE ANY *BUDDHISTS* LIKE US TWO?

I REALLY HAF NO IDEA.

...*PISSES ME OFF!*

STAYING IN A HOTEL WITH MONEY YOU STOLE FROM SOMEONE...

VELL, GUESS THIS IS IT.

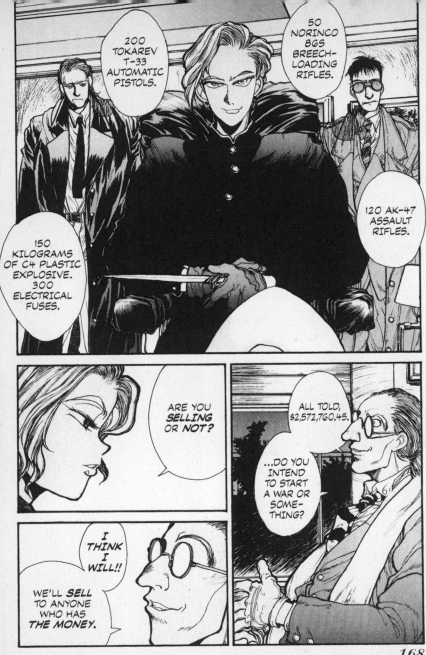

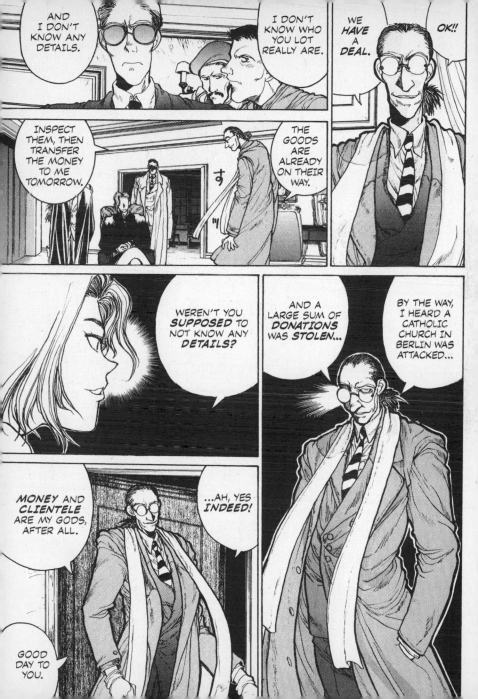

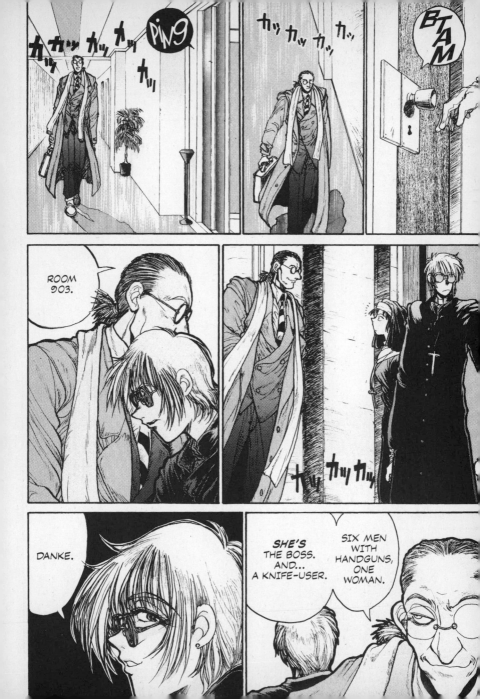

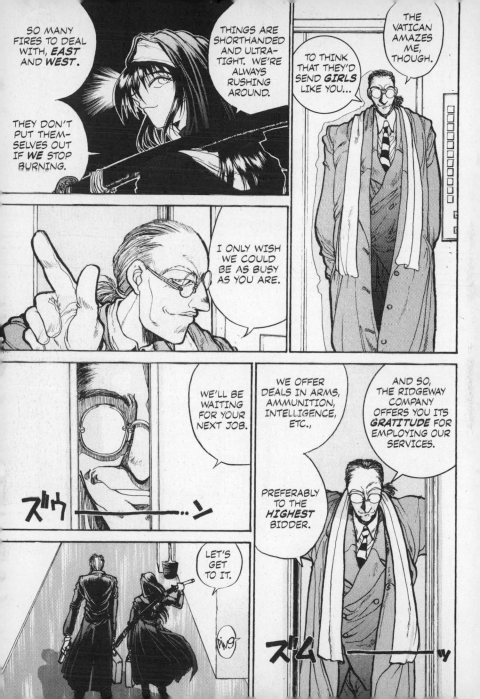

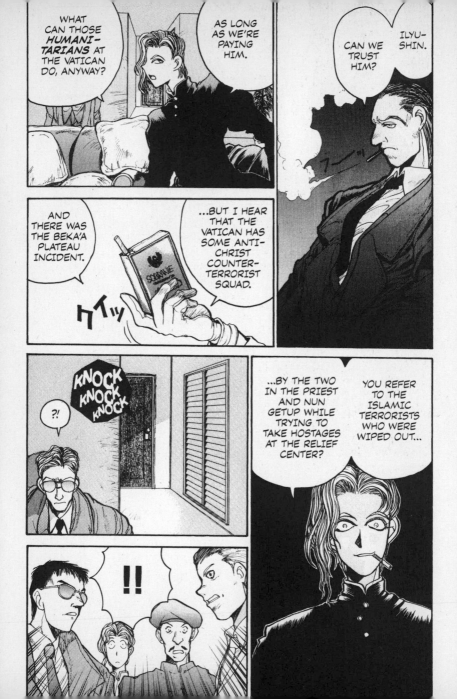

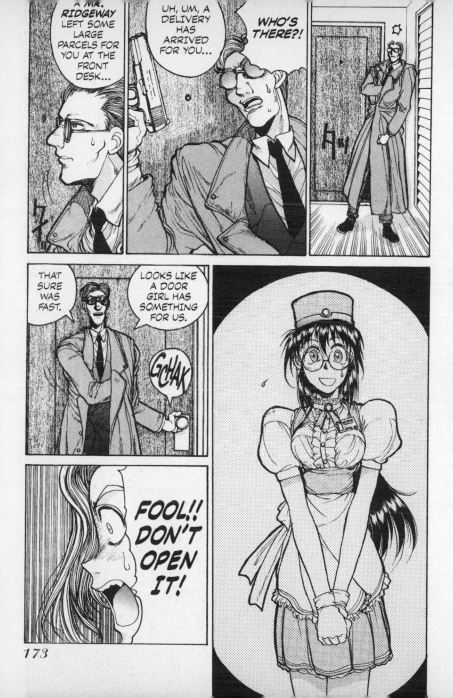

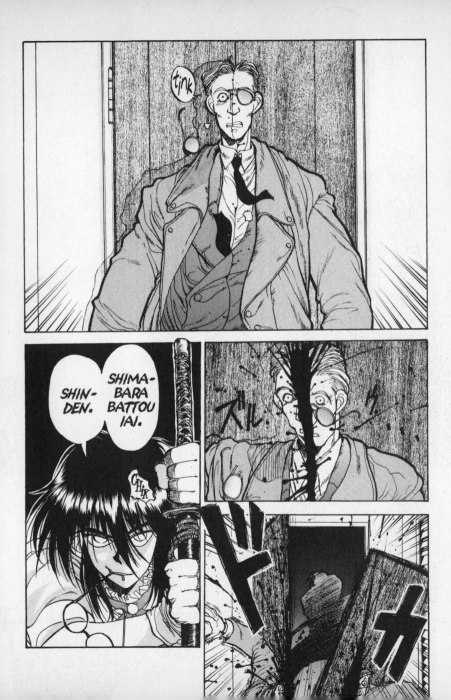

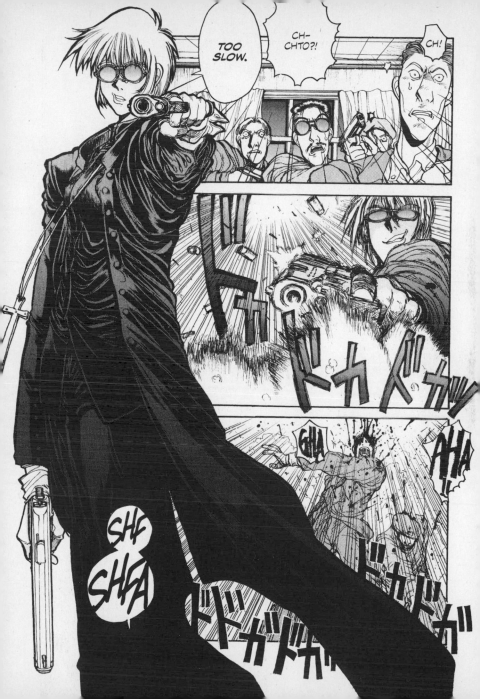

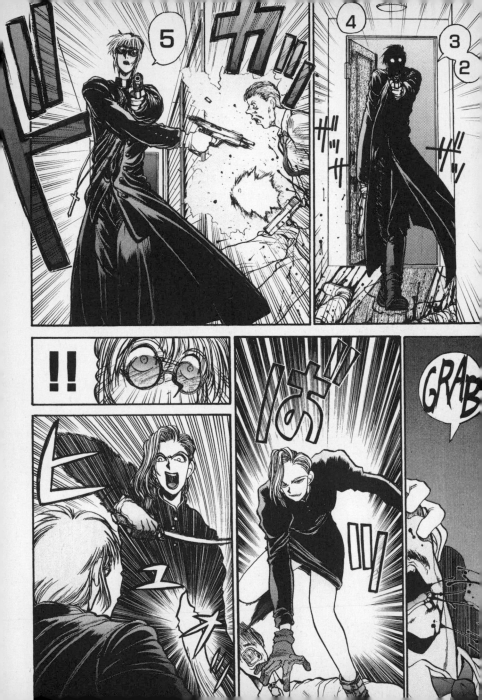

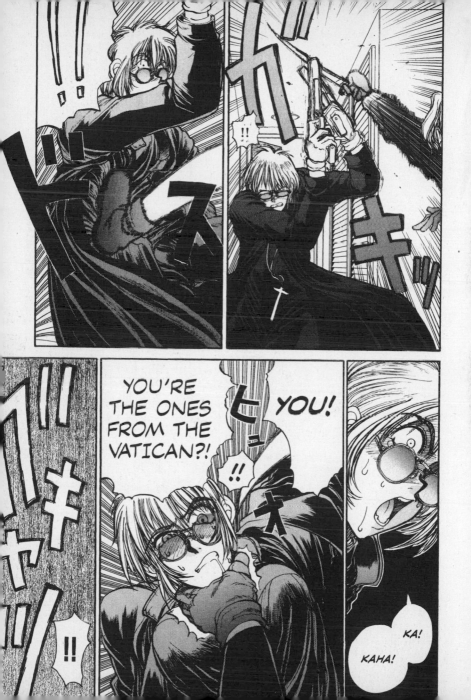

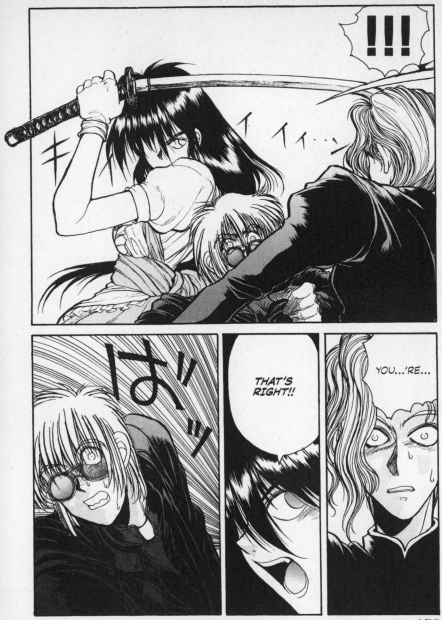

178

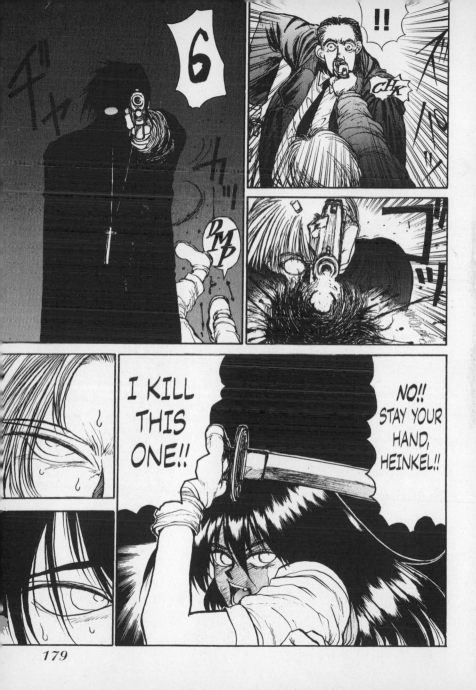

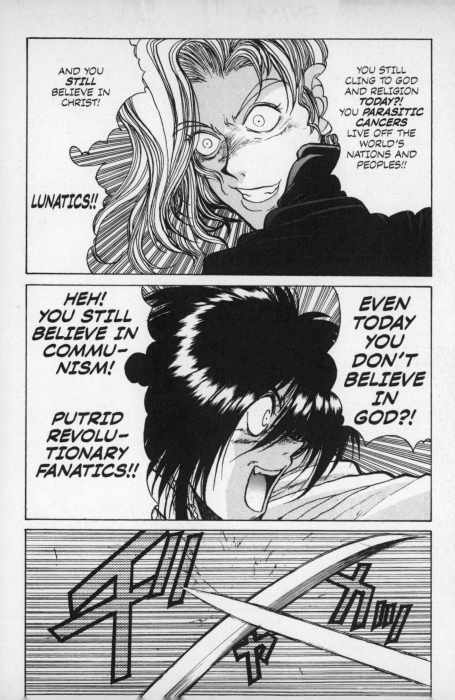

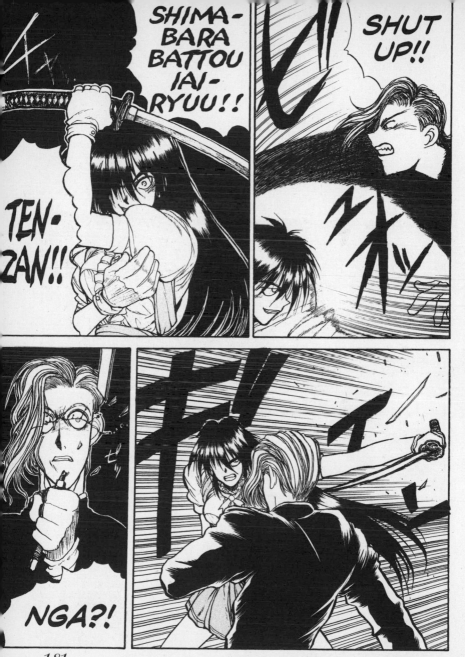

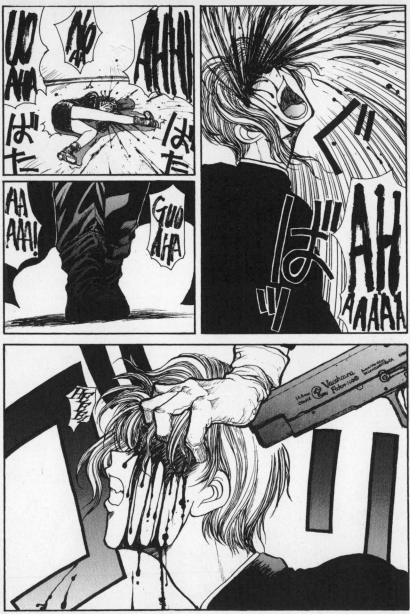

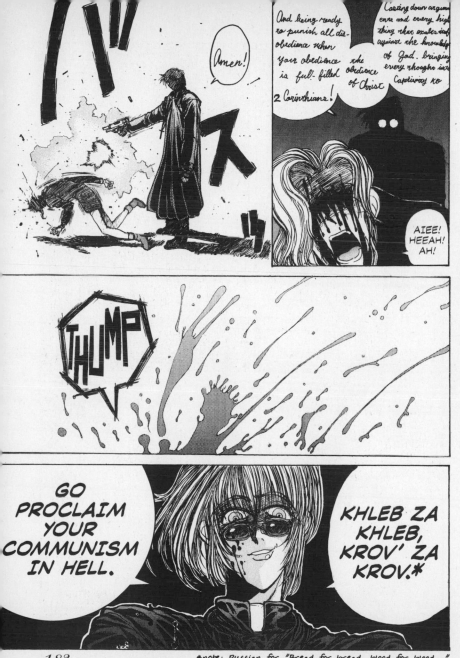

*note: Russian for "Bread for bread, blood for blood..."

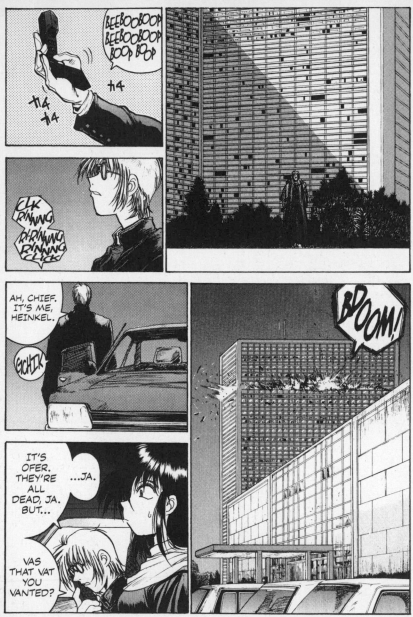

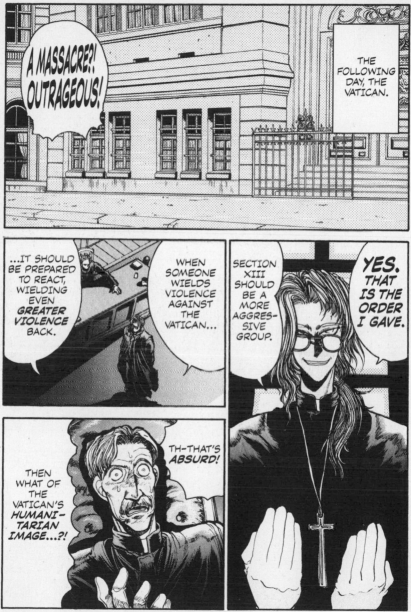

THE FOLLOWING DAY, THE VATICAN.

A MASSACRE?! OUTRAGEOUS!

...IT SHOULD BE PREPARED TO REACT, WIELDING EVEN *GREATER VIOLENCE* BACK.

WHEN SOMEONE WIELDS VIOLENCE AGAINST THE VATICAN...

SECTION XIII SHOULD BE A MORE AGGRESSIVE GROUP.

YES. THAT IS THE ORDER I GAVE.

TH-THAT'S *ABSURD!*

THEN WHAT OF THE VATICAN'S *HUMANITARIAN IMAGE...?!*

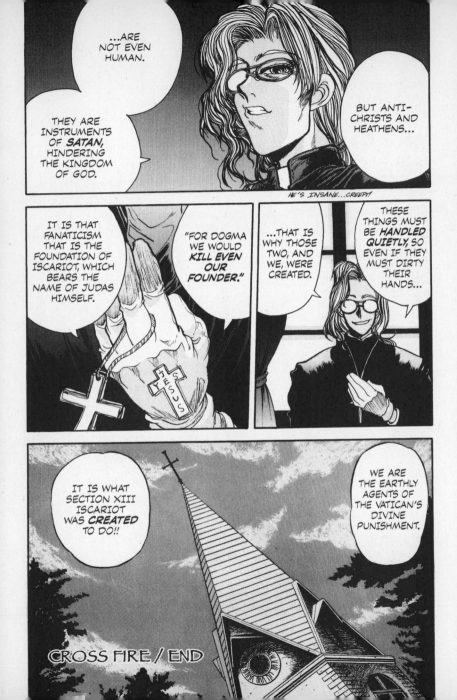

CROSS FIRE / END

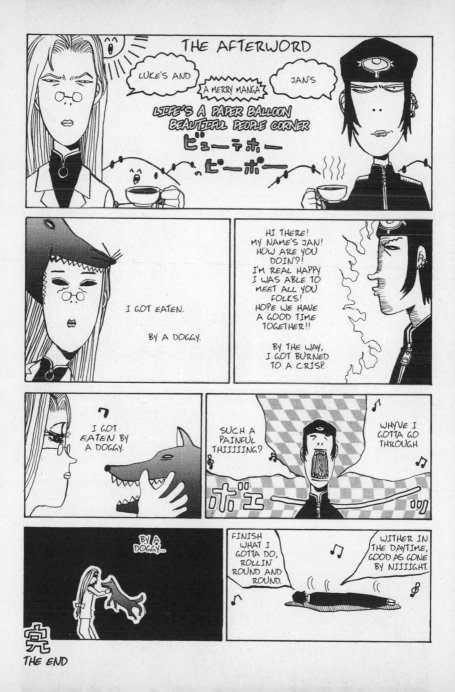

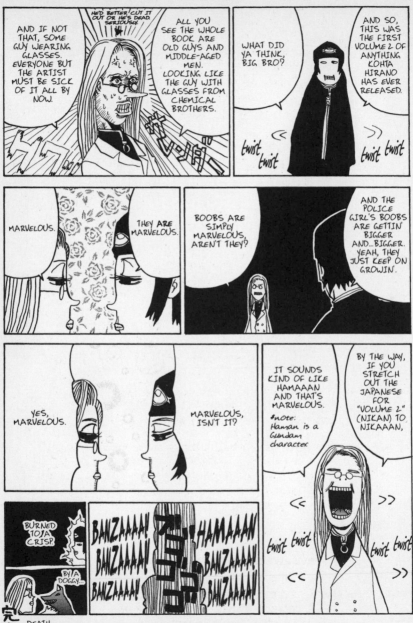

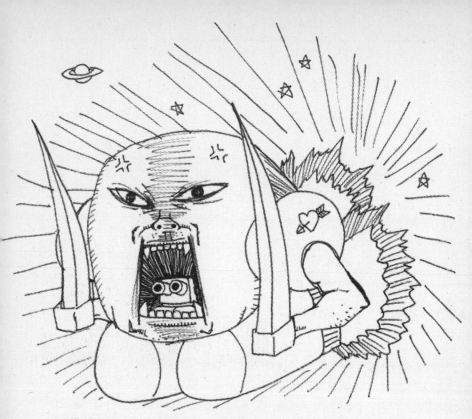

*note: The Zakrello was one of the first models of mobile armor developed in *Mobile Suit Gundam*.

HAILING FROM ADACHI WARD, TOKYO

HOBBY = HARASSMENT, CHINKO IJIRI, BEING ANNOYING, BEATING OFF.
FAVORITE SPACE FORTRESS = A BAOA QU.
note: This is another Gundam reference.

OBNOXIOUS FAVORITE OJAMAJO? = HAZUKI.
note: This refers to the anime Ojamajo Hazuki.

FAVORITE WRESTLER? = HANAYAMA. GRAPPLER.
note: Once again an anime reference. This time it's to Grappler Baki.

FAVORITE NEWTYPE? = HAMAN KARN
note: Yet another Gundam reference.

WHAT DO YOU WANT TO BE IN YOUR NEXT INCARNATION? = MAHARAJA
KARN, THEN GIVE BIRTH TO HAMAN.
note: I don't think I even need to explain at this point.

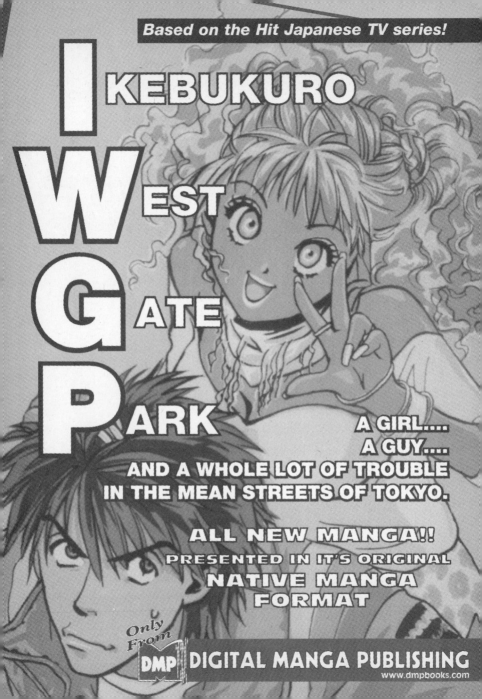

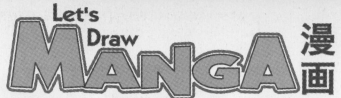

Let's Draw MANGA 漫画

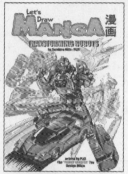
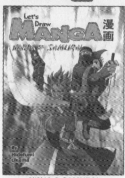
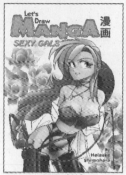
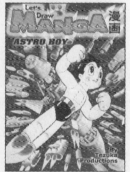
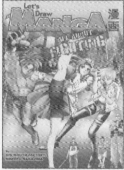
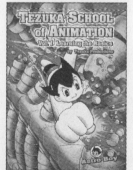
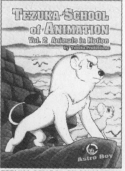
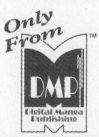

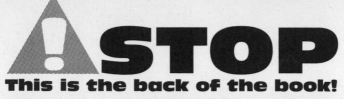

⚠ STOP

This is the back of the book!

This manga collection is translated into English but oriented in right-to-left reading format at the creator's request, maintaining the artwork's visual orientation as originally published in Japan. If you've never read manga in this way before, take a look at the diagram below to give yourself an idea of how to go about it. Basically, you'll be starting in the upper right corner and will read each balloon and panel moving right to left. It may take some getting used to, but you should get the hang of it very quickly. Have fun!

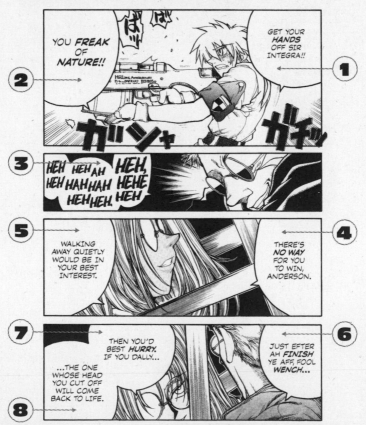